Crop Nutrition:
Principle and Practice

Edited & Compiled By

V.K. Bansal

Educational Publishers & Distributors
291, Bank Enclave, Laxmi Nagar, Delhi-110092.

Published by:

Educational Publishers & Distributors

291, Bank Enclave, Laxmi Nagar, Delhi-110092.

Ph.: (O) 011-65190343, 43551324, 42564726
(M) 9811088729, (Fax) 42564726, (Res.) 47091605

E-mail: *khelsahitya1@rediffmail.com*

Web: *www.khelsahitya.com*

I.S.B.N. - 978-93-80873-45-9

PRINTED IN INDIA 2011

Laser Typeset by:

JAIN MEDIA GRAPHICS

Delhi-110035.

Printed by:

ASIAN OFFSET PRINTERS

Delhi

Price: Rs. 700/-

Contents

in plants and animals, and genomics, nongovernmental organizations, farmers' organizations in developing countries, and private-sector partnerships. The Future Harvest Centers involved in the Biofortification Challenge Program are world renowned for their plant breeding expertise and extensive germplasm banks, strong ties to national agricultural extension programs, and links to the human nutrition community. Thus, they are well placed to coordinate the proposed activities. However, close collaboration with institutions that offer complementary scientific expertise, skills, and experience not found within the Future Harvest Centers, is critical to a successful outcome. To achieve the goals and objectives of the Program, new ways of working together, both within the CGIAR system and with external partners, are needed. Such arrangements are possible under the Challenge Program framework but not under a Systemwide Initiative.

Advantages of Biofortification

The biofortification strategy seeks to take advantage of the consistent daily consumption of large amounts of food staples by all family members, including women and children who are most at risk for micronutrient malnutrition. As a consequence of the predominance of food staples in the diets of the poor, this strategy implicitly targets low-income households. After the one-time investment is made to develop seeds that fortify themselves, recurrent costs are low and germplasm may be shared internationally. It is this multiplier aspect of plant breeding across time and distance that makes it so cost-effective.

Once in place, the biofortified crop system is highly sustainable. Nutritionally improved varieties will continue to be grown and consumed year after year, even if government attention and international funding for micronutrient issues fades.

Biofortification provides a truly feasible means of reaching malnourished populations in relatively remote rural areas, delivering naturally fortified foods to people with limited access commercially-marketed fortified foods, which are more readily available in urban areas. Biofortification and commercial fortification, therefore, are highly complementary.

Breeding for higher trace mineral density in seeds will not incur a yield penalty. In fact, biofortification may have important spinoff effects for increasing farm productivity in developing countries in an environmentally-beneficial way. Mineral-packed seeds sell themselves to farmers because, as recent research has shown, these trace minerals are essential in helping plants resist disease and other environmental stresses. More seedlings survive and initial growth is more rapid. Ultimately, yields are higher, particularly in trace mineral "deficient" soils in arid regions.

Feasibility Studies Support An Expanded Global Research Program

Since 1995, scientists from four Future Harvest Centers of the Consultative Group on International Agricultural Research and partner organizations have been evaluating the feasibility of using modern breeding techniques to produce new varieties of staple crops with high zinc, iron, and betacarotene content. Results to date suggest that biofortification is highly feasible. For most crops, scientists will be able to increase micronutrient densities through conventional breeding by a multiple of two for iron and zinc and by higher multiples for beta-carotene. At the end of this six-year pilot study, scientists agree that the biofortification strategy is feasible 1 but that an expanded global research program is necessary to have the desired impact.

The Biofortification Program will focus on three micronutrients that are widely recognized by the World Health Organization as limiting iron, zinc, and vitamin A. Full-time breeding programs are proposed for six staple foods for which feasibility studies have already been completed and which are consumed by the majority of the world's poor in Africa, Asia, and Latin America: rice, wheat, maize, cassava, sweet potatoes, and common beans. Pre-breeding feasibility studies are proposed for eleven additional staples: bananas, barley, cowpeas, groundnuts, lentils, millet, pigeon peas, plantains, potatoes, sorghum, and yams.

Breeding, dissemination, and impact activities, outlined in the ten-year plan, are focused on development of conventionally-bred crops. No activities involving the release of nutritionally-improved transgenic crops to farmers and consumers are proposed here or are included in proposal budgets for the initial four years for which funding is being requested. Research and development activities with respect to transgenic crops are confined to agricultural research centers and research laboratories. Transgenic methods hold great promise for improving the nutrient content of staple foods and speeding up the breeding process over what can be achieved using conventional methods. High social benefit and lower risk applications, such as the incorporation of desirable traits from crop wild relatives, will be favored throughout the program whenever transgenic methods are considered.

Program Governance and Oversight

A governance and oversight mechanism, led by CIAT and IFPRI, is intended to facilitate these more complex collaborative arrangements. A joint venture or similar agreement will clearly define how CIAT and IFPRI work together and how they will manage the Program. An external, inter-disciplinary Program

Advisory Committee of experts from developing and developed countries is being formed to recommend strategic research priorities, oversee project progress, and implement a transparent competitive grants process. Although the PAC will not be a legal entity, it will have the authority of the CIAT and IFPRI Boards to undertake its mandate as an independent body. A program leader, a breeding and biotechnology coordinator, and a nutrition coordinator, comprising a three-person Program Management Team, will coordinate the overall project and assist the PAC in carrying out its responsibilities. Program activities will be organized by crop, under crop team leaders responsible for coordination.

Regional and cross-crop coordination will be facilitated by the PMT and the relevant crop team leaders.

Extent and Underlying Cause of Micronutrient Malnutrition

Billions of people in developing countries suffer from an insidious form of hunger known as micronutrient malnutrition. Even mild levels of micronutrient malnutrition may damage cognitive development, lower disease resistance in children, and reduce the likelihood that mothers survive childbirth. The costs of these deficiencies in terms of lives lost and poor quality of life are staggering.

It is important to identify who the malnourished are, where they are located, and what they eat in order to develop an effective strategy to reduce micronutrient malnutrition. We know, for example, that they are mostly women and children whose nutritional requirements are highest due to reproduction and rapid growth, who reside in developing countries where dietary quality is often poor.

Extent of Micronutrient Malnutrition

More than 2 billion people worldwide are iron-deficient. Iron deficiency anemia is by far the most common micronutrient deficiency in the world. Iron deficiency during childhood and adolescence impairs physical growth, mental development, and learning capacity. In adults, iron deficiency anemia reduces the capacity to do physical labor. Iron deficiency increases the risk of women dying during delivery or in the postpartum period.

Though these figures also represent anemia brought on by infections, illness, and genetic factors, iron deficiency is by far the most important cause of anemia. Prevalence among children exceeds 50 percent in South and Southeast Asia, where 1.8 billion out of the approximately 4.5 billion people in developing countries live. Prevalence is equally high in Africa, although the number of persons affected is smaller. Prevalence is consistently highest for pregnant women and consistently lowest for adult males

Zinc deficiencies have equally serious consequences for health. For example, meta-analyses of recent randomized controlled trials show that zinc supplementation can reduce morbidity from a number of common childhood infections, especially diarrhea, pneumonia, and possibly malaria, by one-third. In addition, zinc deficiency is an important cause of stunting.

Billions of people are also *at risk for* zinc deficiency. As for anemia, prevalence is highest for South and Southeast Asia and Afric a. Because there is no widely accepted method for measuring of zinc deficiency, no estimates are available of numbers of people who are zinc deficient. Globally, approximately 3 million preschool-age children have visible eye damage owing to vitamin A deficiency. Annually, an estimated 250,000 to 500,000 preschool children go blind from this deficiency, and about two-thirds of these children die within months of going blind. Even more importantly, the last two decades have brought an awareness that vitamin A is essential for immune function. Estimates of the prevalence of subclinical vitamin A deficiency range between 100 million and 250 million for preschool children. People with subclinical vitamin A deficiency more often experience anemia, impaired linear growth, and morbidity from common childhood infections such as respiratory and diarrheal diseases, measles and malaria.

Most importantly, a number of randomized controlled trials in developing countries have shown that administration of vitamin A capsules among infants and preschool children helps reduce mortality rates from all causes by 23 percent and that administration of capsules with vitamin A and beta-carotene among women during childbearing years can reduce maternal mortality related to pregnancy by 40 percent and 49 percent, respectively. Prevalence of vitamin A deficiencies by region is available only for preschool children. Again, similar to iron and zinc, prevalence is highest in South and Southeast Asia and Sub-Saharan Africa.

Underlying Cause of Micronutrient Malnutrition

The primary underlying cause of micronutrient malnutrition is poor quality diets, characterized by high intakes of food staples, but low consumption of animal and fish products, fruits, lentils, and vegetables, which are rich sources of bioavailable minerals and vitamins. As such, most of the malnourished are those who cannot afford to purchase high-quality, micronutrient-rich foods or who cannot obtain these foods from their own production.

Animal and fish products are dense sources of bioavailable micronutrients that the poor wish to eat but cannot afford in large quantities. They account for 25 percent of total food expenditures but only 3 percent of total energy. Nonstaple plant foods such as fruits, vegetables, and lentils are also rich sources of vitamins and minerals. Together, nonstaple plant foods and animal and fish products account for only 20 percent of total energy intakes but 60 percent of food expenditures.

What is perhaps most alarming, however, is the upward trend in nonstaple food prices. Cereal prices have fallen by 40 percent since the early 1970s. The Green Revolution can rightly take credit for its crucial contribution to this tremendous achievement. Falling cereal prices have not only led to increased food security in terms of energy, but also allowed greater purchases of nonstaples by freeing up cash. Unfortunately, however, the rate of production of nonstaple foods has not kept pace with demand, so that these micronutrient-rich food sources have become increasingly expensive for the poor.

Challenge Program Scope and Objectives

The ultimate goal of the biofortification strategy is to reduce mortality and morbidity rates related to micronutrient ma lnutrition and to increase food security, productivity, and the quality of life for poor populations of developing countries by breeding staple crops that provide, at low cost, improved levels of bioavailable micronutrients in a fashion sustainable over time. Developing plant breeding tools, crossing, testing various lines for nutritional effects, eventual dissemination of nutritionally improved varieties, and measuring their effectiveness in reducing malnutrition, indeed putting in place a new paradigm for agriculture and nutrition—is a process that will take a decade. Some intermediate outputs, however, can be made available in a 3- to 5-year time period.

Funding is being sought for a 4-year project that is part of a 10-year plan. At the end of 4 years, it will be possible to evaluate progress and the viability of further investments in the 10-year plan. The 10-year plan is described below, and outputs of the first 4-year project are identified within that plan. The primary objectives of the 10-year plan are to:

- Select and breed nutritionally improved varieties of six major staple food crops with superior agronomic properties that make them attractive to farmers to grow;
- Demonstrate convincingly in the short to medium term the nutritional efficacy of the biofortification strategy;
- Develop efficient, accelerated mechanisms for testing materials on farms, including in areas among the most nutritionally disadvantaged, in order to identify varieties with superior agronomic, socioeconomic, and farmer-acceptable traits;
- Undertake activities to promote the adoption and dissemination of these varieties efficiently and rapidly in selected developing countries in Africa, Asia, and Latin America among the nutritionally disadvantaged; and
- Measure the nutritional and other impacts of these nutritionally improved varieties in communitybased studies where these varieties have been adopted.

Complementary objectives are to:

- Initiate prebreeding studies to determine the feasibility of undertaking full-scale breeding programs for an additional eleven food staple crops;
- Understand better how dietary factors determine the bioavailability of micronutrients in malnourished populations in developing countries, especially interactions among micronutrients, anti-nutrients such as phytates, promoter compounds, and physiological status; and
- Inform decisionmakers in developing countries about cost-effective strategies to reduce micronutrient malnutrition through food-based approaches and policies to improve dietary quality among the poor.

Staple food crops under the project are classified into two groups:

- Phase 1 crops, for which the knowledge base already exists to breed for improved micronutritional quality: wheat, maize, rice, sweet potatoes, common beans, and cassava; and
- Phase 2 crops, for which the knowledge base must be established: sorghum, millet, groundnuts, pigeon peas, lentils, barley, cowpeas, yams, potatoes, bananas, and plantains.

The primary target micronutrient deficiencies are iron, zinc, and vitamin A. Delivery of improved, biofortified varieties to end-users will be assured through an alliance of international centers, NARES, ARIs, NGOs, and farmers' organizations and the use of participatory breeding techniques. As already stated, the biofortification breeding strategy is envisioned as a complement to other successful ongoing approaches, including supplementation and fortification.

Why a Challenge Program

The Biofortification Challenge Program pushes the

boundaries of agricultural research beyond the traditional limits of food security and sustainability and makes direct linkages with the human health and nutrition sectors. By making a formal connection between what people grow and consume and how healthy they are as a result, the program marries the often separate agendas of the international nutrition and agricultural research communities in the context of working concertedly to address a specific problem of global concern: micronutrient malnutrition.

This linkage of agricultural research and human health goals raises the profile of the international agricultural research system and gives new relevance to the often unheralded work being done throughout the CGIAR-supported Future Harvest centers and our partners in the developing and developed world. Building on a solid foundation of research results, the program will develop, deploy, and measure the nutritional impact of micronutrient-improved varieties of staple crops consumed by the poorest of the poor in Africa, Asia, and Latin America.

Activities will be undertaken by an international alliance of Future Harvest Centers, national agricultural research and extension systems departments of human nutrition and plant science at universities in developing and developed countries, advanced research institutes with expertise in micronutrients in plants and animals, and genomics, nongovernmental organizations, farmers' organizations in developing countries, and private-sector partnerships. The Future Harvest Centers involved in the Biofortification Challenge Program are world renowned for their plant breeding expertise and extensive germplasm banks, strong ties to national agricultural extension programs, and links to the human nutrition community. Thus, they are well placed to coordinate the proposed activities. However, close collaboration with institutions that offer complementary scientific expertise, skills, and experience not found within the Future Harvest Centers is critical to a successful outcome. To achieve the goals and objectives of the Program, new ways of working together, both within the

CGIAR system and with external partners, are needed. Such arrangements are possible under the Challenge Program framework but not under a Systemwide Initiative. There are significant advantages to working together in a coordinated fashion, under the rubric of a challenge program:

- Program success depends critically on the alignment of objectives and the coordinated efforts of institutions with diverse disciplinary perspectives, experience, and skills.
- These multiple partnerships, many formed with nontraditional collaborators of the CGIAR system, require strong central coordination to avoid loss of program focus.
- Interdisciplinary communication within single crop activities and common experiences across these crop activities will stimulate fresh insights and discovery of novel solutions.
- Standardization of methodologies (such as sample analyses) will lead to greater acceptance and applicability of results.
- Program-coordinated work in nutritional genomics, identification of breeding objectives, and other core research applicable across crops or nutrients will avoid duplication of efforts and result in cost savings.

When topsoil dries, roots in the dry soil zone which are easiest to fertilize are largely deactivated and the plant must rely on deep roots for further nutrition. Roots of plant genotypes that are efficient in mobilizing surrounding, ext ernal trace minerals, are not only more disease resistant, but also better able to penetrate deficient subsoils, and so make use of the moisture and minerals contained in subsoils. This reduces the need for fertilizers and improves drought tolerance.

In addition, fewer herbicides and pesticides would have

to be used because micronutrient-efficient genotypes should have greater resistance to plant pathogens.

These characteristics benefit those whose soils are deficient in trace minerals on rainfed land and who are thus among the poorest farmers.

- Consolidation of the main advocacy, fund-raising, communications, and other administrative burdens will permit the individual partners to focus on the core research, development, deployment, and impact analysis activities.
- Attraction of new sources of funding is best handled through centralized coordination. The program will heighten the profile of the CGIAR system as an important world body addressing pressing global concerns.

Biofortification: A New Tool to Reduce Micronutrient Malnutrition

Modern agriculture has had reasonable success in meeting the energy needs of developing countries. In the past 40 years, agricultural research in developing countries has met Malthus' challenge by placing increased cereal production at its center. However, agriculture must now focus on a new paradigm that will not only produce more food, but bring us better quality food as well.

By producing staple foods whose edible portions are more dense in bioavailable minerals and vitamins, a process referred to here as "biofortification," scientists can provide farmers with crop varieties that naturally reduce anemia, cognitive impairment, and other nutritionally related health problems in hundreds of millions of people. Biofortification can provide an additional instrument in the fight to reduce micronutrient malnutrition, one that uses food as a mechanism to improve human health. The CGIAR Biofortification Challenge Program will focus on improving the nutritional content of the staple foods poor people already eat, providing a comparatively inexpensive, cost-effective, sustainable, long-term means of delivering micronutrients to the poor. This approach will not only lower the number of severely malnourished people who require treatment by complementary interventions, but also will help maintain an improved nutritional status. Moreover, biofortification provides a feasible means of reaching malnourished populations, especially in rural areas, with limited access to supplements or commercially marketed fortified foods.

Unlike the continual financial outlays required for traditional supplementation and fortification programs, a one-time investment in breeding-based solutions can yield micronutrient-rich plants for farmers to grow around the world for years to come. It is this multiplier aspect of biofortification across time and distance that makes it so cost-effective.

The Potential Impact of Biofortification on Micronutrient Malnutrition

No single type of intervention can by itself solve the micronutrient malnutrition problem. A comprehensive strategy involving multiple types of interventions adapted to conditions in specific countries and regions is required. The final, permanent solution to micronutrient malnutrition in developing countries is a substantial improvement in dietary quality higher consumption of pulses, fruits, vegetables, fish, and animal products, which the poor already desire but cannot presently afford.

Meanwhile, breeding staple foods that are dense in minerals and vitamins provides a low-cost, sustainable strategy for reducing levels of micronutrient malnutrition. Biofortification complements existing strategies and has its own unique "niche," as conditioned by the comparative advantages outlined above and technical characteristics, most importantly the level of the "dose" that biofortification can be expected. An important part of the overall solution is to improve the productivity of a long list of nonstaple food crops.

Because of the large number of foods involved, achieving this goal requires a very large investment, the dimensions of which are not addressed here. On any given day, biofortified staple foods cannot deliver as high a level of minerals and vitamins as supplements or industrially fortified foods, but they can help to bring millions over the threshold from malnourishment to micronutrient suffic iency. For those who are severely deficient, supplements the highest-cost intervention are required. Commercial fortification and biofortification lower-cost, lower-"dose" strategies then are highly complementary, in at least two ways, in treating the bulk of the iron-deficient population. First, there is a time dimension. Commercial fortification is a proven intervention and already being implemented. If the activities under the Biofortification Challenge Program proceed successfully, gradually those being reached by biofortified crops will reduce the need for commercial fortification. Second, there is a

Potential to Reduce Iron and Zinc Deficiency

Poor consumers in developing countries acquire roughly one-half of their total iron intake and a higher percentage of zinc intake from staple foods. Results from germplasm screening suggest that the iron and zinc content of staple foods can be doubled through conventional breeding. This result, in turn, implies that iron and zinc intakes in poor people's diets can be increased by 50 percent. This should result in an appreciable improvement in nutrition and health even for those whose intakes remain below recommended daily intakes.

No adverse effects other than carotenodermia a harmless yellow coloration of the skin have been reported from very high consumption of beta-carotene or other carotenoids in foods. Beta-carotene is used therapeutically, at extremely high doses approximately 180 mg per day, for the treatment of erythropoietic protoporphyria, a photosensitivity disorder. No toxic side effects have been observed at these doses. There is no evidence that betacarotene or other carotenoids are teratogenic, mutagenic, or carcinogenic in long-term bioassays in experimental animals. In addition, long-term supplementation with beta-carotene to persons with adequate vitamin A status does not increase the concentration of serum retinol. country population, this increased iron intake would reduce anemia prevalence by about 5 percent among populations consuming iron-biofortified food staples, say from 50 percent to 45 percent.

As more is learned, for example, about genes that control iron transport in plants and iron-loading into seeds and about compounds that promote mineral bioavailability, it should be possible in the future to substantially upgrade these conservative estimates of the drop in iron-deficiency prevalences that could be effected through biofortification. A more reasonable expectation might be a 10–20 percent reduction in prevalence say from 40 percent prevalence to a 20–30 percent prevalence among consuming populations.

Consider a future scenario in which iron-biofortified crops are being consumed by 25 percent of the population in developing countries and where anemia prevalences fall by 10 percent among consuming populations. More than 100 million cases of iron-deficiency could be averted each year.

As compared with analysis undertaken above for iron, far less is known about levels of zinc intakes, prevalence of zinc deficiency, and the relationship between zinc intakes and zinc deficiency. As for iron, germplasm screening under the CGIAR Micronutrients Project suggests that zinc density can be increased substantially through conventional breeding, perhaps by 100% in rice and wheat and by 75% in beans. The data in Box 2 for rural Bangladesh for which some information is available on zinc intakes, indicate that rice is an even more predominant source of zinc than of iron in the low quality diets of the poor. This, in turn, suggests that a larger impact might be made on zinc intakes than on iron intakes.

Potential Impact of Zinc-dense Food Staples on Zinc Intakes

The table below shows the high contribution of rice to total zinc intakes in rural Bangladesh compared with the contribution of rice to total iron intakes. If the zinc density of milled rice can be doubled from 11 to 22 mg kg, this would result in a 70 percent increase in zinc intakes. An increment of 8 mg/kg of iron in milled rice would add 4 milligrams of iron per day to the intakes of females. See Gregorio (2001) for estimates of the range of genetic variation available for iron and zinc in rice.

The Potential to Reduce Vitamin A Deficiency

The geographic areas of largest potential impact are those subregions of Africa and Latin America where 7 Due to the presence in staple grains of anti-nutrient compounds, only a fraction of this iron will be absorbed and become available for physiological processes in the human body.

Potential Impact of Biofortification on Agronomic Productivity and Farm Costs

Good nutrition balance is as important to disease resistance and stress tolerance in plants as it is in humans. Micronutrient deficiency in plants greatly increases their susceptibility to diseases, especially fungal root diseases of the major food crops. Efficiency in the uptake of mineral micronutrients from the soil is associated with disease resistance in plants, which leads to decreased use of fungicides. Breeding for micronutrient efficiency can confer resistance to root diseases that had previously been unattainable. Micronutrient-efficient varieties grow deeper roots in mineral-deficient soils and are better at tapping subsoil water and minerals. When topsoil dries, roots in the dry soil zone which are the easiest to fertilize are largely deactivated and the plant must rely on deeper roots for further nutrition. Roots of plant genotypes that are efficient in mobilizing surrounding external minerals not only are more disease resistant, but are better able to penetrate deficient subsoils and so make use of the moisture and minerals contained in subsoils. This reduces the need for fertilizers and irrigation. Plants with deeper root systems are more drought resistant.

A soil is said to be deficient in a given nutrient when the

addition of fertilizer produces better growth even though the amount of nutrient in the fertilizer added may be small compared with the total amount of the nutrient in the soil. This seeming paradox can occur when only a small part of the nutrient in the soil is available to plants, owing, for example, to the chemical properties of the soil. Alternatively, the view can be taken that there is a genetic deficiency in the plant rather than a deficiency in the soil. Rather than adapting the soil to the plant, breeding can adapt the plant to the soil.

The table below gives an analysis of both total and extractable micronutrients in one trace element-deficient sandy soil in comparison with the nutrients removed in the grain of an average crop grown on that soil. The picture presented for nitrogen is quite different from that for trace minerals. Few soils of the world can sustain high yields for long periods without additional supplies of nitrogen, either by rotation of the crop with nitrogenfixing legumes or from mineral fertilizer additions. Thus, it is pointless to breed for greater tolerance to nitrogendeficient soils. Trace minerals are present in much greater concentrations compared with plant needs even in a nutrient-impoverished soil such as that below. It is logical, then, to concentrate breeding efforts on these elements with low requirements or low availability, but large reserves in the soil.

A significant percentage of the soils in which staple foods are grown are "deficient" in these trace minerals, which has kept crop yields low. In general, these soils, in fact, contain high amounts of trace minerals, enough for hundreds or thousands of crops. However, because of chemical binding to other compounds, these trace minerals are "unavailable" to staple crop varieties presently used.

Depletion of soils of trace minerals may never occur at all, owing to various inadvertent additions such as windblown dust. Therefore, the traits of efficient uptake of trace minerals from the soil and of loading of those trace minerals into the seed are compatible with breeding for high yields. Farmers can be expected to adopt genotypes with trace mineral-dense seeds out of a profit motive. High-mineral seed density is compatible with high yields; this trait can be incorporated into the best-yielding varieties. In Bangladesh and India, approximately 80 million hectares are sown to rice and wheat each year. Suppose that 25 percent of this land (20 million hectares is sown to iron- and zinc-dense varieties and that the seed zinc density imparts an increase in yield of 250 kg hectare of unmilled rice and wheat on 8 million hectares 40 percent of the 20 million hectares. This increase in yield, with a value of perhaps US$35 per hectare, times 8 million hectares, would give a benefit of US$280 million per year.

In addition, Cakmak et al. has estimated that seeding rates for zinc-efficient wheat genotypes on 5 million hectares of zinc-"deficient" soils in Turkey can be lowered from 250 kg hectares to 170 kg/hectares thanks to greater seedling vigor and vitality. This change would save farmers US$16 per hectare in input costs. On 5 million hectares of land, this represents a savings of US$80 million per year to farmers in Turkey not including the value of increased wheat yields or improved human nutrition.

Comparative Advantages of Biofortification

Eliminating micronutrient malnutrition in any one country will require bringing to bear an array of interventions including supplementation, commercial fortification, and greater dietary diversity through nutrition education and higher incomes. Biofortification must have some comparative advantages relative to existing interventions to justify investments in this approach. These comparative advantages are discussed below.

Reaching the Malnourished in Rural Areas

Modern varieties of crops developed by the CGIAR and NARES and disseminated by NGOs and government extension agencies are grown extensively by poor farmers, even in relatively remote regions. The biofortification strategy seeks to put the micronutrient-dense seed trait in the most profitable, highestyielding varieties being released to farmers by agricultural research systems as many released lines as future research and experience indicates are feasible. Thus, nutritionally improved varieties would reach into relatively remote rural areas not presently well covered by commercial fortification and supplementation programs. Moreover, marketed surpluses of these crops would make their way into retail outlets, reaching consumers in both rural and urban areas. The direction of the flow, as it were, is from rural to urban. Often commercial fortification works best for imported foods such as wheat flour that are processed at a few central industrial establishments. These foods flow from urban to rural locations. This situation clearly shows the complementarity of biofortification and commercial fortification.

Cost-Effectiveness and Low Cost

Unlike the continual financial outlays required for supplementation and fortification programs, a one-time investment in breeding-based solutions can yield micronutrient-rich plants for farmers to grow around the world for years to come. It is this multiplier aspect of biofortification across time and distance that makes it so cost-effective.

In an analysis of commercial fortification, Horton and Ross estimate that the present value of each annual case of iron deficiency averted in South Asia is approximately US$20.9 Consider the value of 1 billion cases of iron deficiency averted in years 16–25 after a biofortification research and development project was initiated. The nominal value of US$20 billion must be discounted because of the lags involved between the time that investments are made in biofortification and when benefits are realized. At a 3 percent discount rate, the present value would be approximately US$10 billion, and at a 12 percent discount rate, the present value would be approximately US$2 billion.

These calculations count no benefit to those with anemia whose iron status improves, as indicated by hemoglobin concentrations, but without crossing the threshold of anemia. Iron-biofortified crops would reach more than 1 billion such iron-deficient people each year, under an assumption of a 25 percent spread of these biofortified varieties in developing countries, or more than 10 billion iron-deficient people over a decade. Biofortified crops would also reach those who are iron-sufficient but whose iron stores would be increased.

If US$150 million in discounted investments were spent on developing, testing, disseminating, and maintaining iron-biofortified food staples, under the above scenario the cost would be 15 cents for each case of iron-deficiency averted US$150 million divided by 100 million cases averted and 1.5 cents for each iron-deficient person reached US$150 million divided by 1 billion iron-deficient people reached.

As a basis of comparison, the cost of commercial fortification is 10 cents per person reached, whether the 9 A World Bank study assigns a present value benefit of US$45 to each annual case of iron deficiency averted through fortification a mix of age-gender groups. The same study gives a present value of US$96 for each annual case of vitamin A deficiency averted for preschoolers.

Because these research and development expenditures are incurred over a decade, these costs need to be discounted as well, say US$10 million in discounted costs per crop. Multiplying by six major staple foods gives US$60 million in discounted costs. Ninety million dollars in discounted costs for extension education are added to give the total figure of US$150 million in discounted costs.

The cost of iron supplementation is US$2 per iron-deficient person reached. High-iron and high-zinc traits appear to be genetically linked. Thus, it should be relatively easy to breed high-iron and high-zinc varieties simultaneously. The calculations above count no benefit to human nutrition of increased zinc intakes or to improved productivity due to higher loading of zinc into seeds. And, of course, the calculations do not count any benefits prior to year 16 or after year 25, even though biofortified varieties would be available before and after these years.

Sustainability of Biofortification

Once in place, the system described in the previous section is highly sustainable. The major, fixed costs of developing the varieties and convincing the nutrition and plant science communities of their importance and effectiveness will have already been borne. Government attention to micronutrient issues may fade. International funding for micronutrient interventions may be substantially reduced. But the nutritionally improved varieties will continue to be grown and consumed year after year. To be sure, recurrent expenditures are required for monitoring and maintaining these traits in crops. But these recurrent costs are low compared with the cost of the initial development of the nutritionally improved crops and the establishment, institutionally speaking, of nutrient content as a bona fide breeding objective.

Behavioral Change

Mineral micronutrients make up a tiny fraction of the physical mass of a seed, 5–10 parts per million in milled rice. Dense bean seeds may contain as many as 100 parts per million. Whether such small amounts will alter the appearance, taste, texture, or cooking quality of foods will need be investigated. If increased densities in iron and zinc are not noticeable by consumers, the dissemination strategy for trace minerals, then, could rely on *existing* producer and consumer behavior. Analogous to the additio n of fluoride to drinking water in some developed countries, successful implementation would not require that farmers and consumers know that they are producing and eating more nutritious varieties, although this information would be publicly advertised and publicly available.

In contrast, higher levels of beta-carotene will turn varieties from white or light colors of yellow to dark yellow and orange.

Often, consumers much prefer white varieties of, for example, milled rice, wheat flour, maize, and cassava. Major nutrition education programs will have to be mounted to encourage consumers t~ switch to more nutritious varieties and incorporated in benefit-cost calculations such as in the previous section. If these nutrition education programs are successful, however, the yellow-orange color will distinguish the more nutritious varieties from the less nutritious and a disadvantage will have been turned into an advantage.

Feasibility of Breeding for Nutritious Crops Demonstrated

The CGIAR Micronutrients Project is an ongoing interdisciplinary effort of plant scientists, human nutritionists, and social scientists. The overall objective of the project has been to evaluate the feasibility of using modern breeding techniques to produce new varieties of staple crops that are eaten by the poor with high micronutrient content. The search for promising germplasm has been conducted in the seed banks of IRRI in the Philippines, the International Center for Tropical Agriculture in Colombia, and the International Center for the Improvement of Maize and Wheat in Mexico. This research, coordinated by the International Food Policy Research Institute has been carried out in collaboration with scientists at the University of Adelaide in Australia and research labs of the United States Department of Agriculture located at Cornell University in Ithaca, New York, and the University of California at Davis.

During the past six years three scientists among the proposed collaborators in nutritional genomics have obtained significant funding from competitively awarded scientific funds to study molecular and genetic aspects of carotenoids and vitamin E synthesis and iron and zinc accumulation mechanisms in plants. This knowledge and expertise will be leveraged in the course of this proposed technology development and deployment project.

Results thus far indicate that biofortification is highly feasible. For most crops, there is adequate genetic variation in concentrations of beta-carotene, other functional carotenoids, iron, zinc, and other trace minerals in varieties available in CGIAR germplasm banks to increase micronutrient densities through conventional breeding by a multiple of two for trace minerals and by higher multiples for beta-carotene. Results also show that:

- Micronutrient density traits are stable across growing environments;
- It is possible to combine the high micronutrient density trait with high yield, unlike protein content and yield, which are negatively correlated;
- Genetic control of target nutritional traits is simple enough to make breeding economical;
- It is possible to improve the content of several micronutrients together in a single variety; and
- Bioavailability of the extra trace minerals in elite breeding lines is high in *in vitro* and animal tests; tests on human populations are now a high priority.

At the end of the pilot phase, scientists agree that the biofortification strategy is feasible 12 but that an expanded global research program is necessary. Third, there are expected to be important synergies in research across crops. It may be that an important discovery for one crop will inform work on other crops as well. Fourth, ignoring dietary diversity and focusing research investments on a small number of widely grown staple foods is arguably responsible in part for the present situation of poor dietary quality. The micronutrient density of as many foods as possible should be increased, starting with the broad range of food staples. In any event, the requested funds for the Phase 2 crops are relatively modest to support studies of the feasibility of undertaking full-scale nutrition breeding programs for these crops.

Research Activities and Methods

The 10-year plan objectives will be accomplished through a series of interdisciplinary activities. The major activities to be undertaken are:

- Plant breeding based at Future Harvest centers and national agricultural research systems for six Phase 1 crops, using a dual approach: early development of "fast-track" varieties that will convincingly demonstrate the validity of the biofortification strategy; and a more lengthy parallel development of varieties combining the best nutritio nal and agronomic traits in each crop, using adaptive decentralized breeding methods and seed production where feasible;
- Prebreeding feasibility studies based at Future Harvest centers for 10 Phase 2 crops important in the diets of those suffering from mic ronutrient deficiencies but for which the knowledge base for biofortification has yet to be developed;
- Initial screening of promising lines for micronutrient bioavailability using *in vitro* and animal models and subsequent efficacy studies involving human subjects to evaluate nutritional impact of the most promising lines intended for release;
- Dissemination of nutritionally improved varieties through collaboration with farmers, NARES, and NGOs, and evaluation of effectiveness of the biofortification strategy after adoption;
- Application of novel advances in genomics, genetics, and molecular biology to identify and understand plant biosynthetic genes and pathways of nutritional importance; use of this knowledge (1) in marker-assisted selection for conventional breeding of Phase 1 crops and (2) in initial development (but not release) of transgenic lines;
- Research to understand economic and social factors that determine the dietary quality of the poor and their

micronutrient status, and policy advocacy based on that research; and

- Coordinated communication activities designed to provide support to internal project constituents and external audiences, including donors, the academic and development communities, public officials, and the general media.

Human Nutrition Activities

University partners will help identify nutritionally optimal breeding strategies and conduct nutrition efficacy trials. Impact studies will involve collaboration among these university partners, social scientists at the relevant Future Harvest centers, and local partners. Analyses related to human nutrition will be conducted in four areas:

- Basic studies will investigate optimal strategies that is, identifying breeding objectives for maximizing nutrient bioavailability through increasing micronutrient density, reducing antinutrients, and or increasing promoter compounds. This work will be initiated by Robin Graham and James Stangoulis at the University of Adelaide and Ross Welch at PSNL on the Cornell University campus.
- The PSNL will undertake *in vitro* and animal studies to provide initial screening of bioavailability for promising genotypes for each crop.
- Midproject efficacy trials involving human subjects to test nutritionally improved lines for each crop will be undertaken in developing countries under the direction of nutritionists from developed-country universities in collaboration with developing-country nutritionists. Areas will be selected in which the prevalent diets are representative of wide geographic regions and in which two or more of the crops under study are staples, thus incorporating the food-system approach.

- In the final phase of the project, once nutritionally improved varieties have been adopted, community-based impact studies will be undertaken by these same teams of nutritionists in selected countries, including an evaluation of the effectiveness of the nutritionally improved varieties in reducing micronutrient malnutrition.

Plant Breeding Activities

Conventional

A recommendation for initiating a full-scale breeding program for the six Phase 1 target crops is based on favorable previous findings summarized in section 2.1. The target micronutrients to be improved are iron, zinc, and beta-carotene. Breeding activities include:

Many other factors influence the degree to which ingested micronutrients are absorbed (bioavailability) and utilized bioefficacy, including a person's micronutrient and health status. Given this complexity, three breeding sub-strategies may be applied individually or in various combinations. These are (1) increasing the mineral and vitamin content, (2) reducing the level of anti-nutrients in food staples that inhibit the bioavailability of minerals and vitamins, and (3) increasing the levels of nutrients and compounds that promote the bioavailability of minerals and vitamins.

For example, phytates and tannins inhibit iron and zinc absorption. Proposed in vitro and animal studies and efficacy feeding trials will evaluate effects of these inhibiting compounds. With respect to compounds that promote bioavailability, certain amino acids (such as cysteine) enhance iron and/or zinc bioavailability. These amino acids occur in many staple foods, but their concentrations are lower than those found in meat products. A modest increase in the concentrations of promoter amino acids in plant foods may have a positive effect on iron and zinc bioavailability in humans. Iron and zinc occur only in micromolar amounts in plant foods, so only micromolar increases in the amounts of these amino acids may be required to compensate for the negative effects of anti-nutrients on iron and zinc bioavailability. These amino acids are essential nutrients for plants as well as for humans, so relatively small increases of their concentrations in plant tissues should not have adverse consequences on plant growth.

While the Biofortification Challenge Program pursues breeding for higher micronutrient content as its initial breeding objective, at the same time an effort will be made to investigate the possibly large nutritional impacts of the extended breeding strategies suggested above. This component of the project explores genetic variation in nutrient content in staple crop plants and the interactions among nutrients in animals and humans that can dictate improved strategies of plant breeding for nutritional quality. The idea is to exploit potential synergies in the human body to simplify the breeding objectives by decreasing the number of genes needed in a breeding program, thereby optimizing the cost-effectiveness of the strategy. The results of the research from this component of the project will inform breeding strategies for all crops.

For a fuller discussion of these topics, see supporting documents on activities to be undertaken in the area of human nutrition which are described.

- Additional germplasm evaluation of materials with potential for short-term impact;
- Implementation of molecular markers for large-scale selection programs;
- Genetic and QTL analyses to determine loci involved in micronutrient content; and
- Development of varieties with high micronutrient concentration and superior agronomic traits, in collaboration with NARES and farmers' groups.

Breeding has been the strength of the CGIAR centers since

their inception, as a logical extension of the gene banks that are held in the centers. For every crop listed in this project, significant success has been obtained in the areas of disease resistance, tolerance to abiotic stresses and or yield potential. Productivity of several crops has been increased dramatically, and these objectives continue to be important as breeders look to the future.

From this perspective, can breeders assume still another breeding objective? Breeders involved in this project do not feel that this is unrealistic. The experience in IRRI's rice program suggests that a moderate level of iron was achieved even without directed screening in a few modern varieties. This modest success can be greatly amplified by breeding consciously and systematically for higher micronutrients, thus exploiting opportunities that have been observed in the germplasm where much greater levels are to be found.

"Conventional" breeding is made even more efficient by integrating a set of tools such as: markerassisted selection for key agronomic and nutritional traits; molecular biology for gene discovery of relevant traits; and transgenics to increase existing levels or provide opportunities that are lacking within the respective crop species.

In the final analysis, the requirement is that 3-4 genes be added to the suite of genes that breeders successfully work with in their breeding programs. This is tota lly feasible with the tools described above, and breeders feel comfortable that they can increase levels of micronutrients while continuing to make gains in agronomic breeding objectives. Materials to be released will have superior agronomic traits to facilitate adoption by farmers. QPM maize is now fully competitive with standard maize varieties and often out yields these, making them attractive to producers. Biofortified maize will build on progress in QPM and expand these successes to higher levels of iron and zinc. Progress has been registered in beans for superior drought tolerance and this in turn will be the basis for new varieties with better nutritional quality. Results for several crops show that there is no penalty in yield or other traits from increasing micronutrient content.

Nutritional Genomics Activities

Nutritional genomics is a new approach to the study of complex biochemical pathways in plants. It seeks to elucidate the basic, underlying mechanisms involved in the synthesis and accumulation of essential vitamins and minerals in plant tissues. Because of the metabolic unity among organisms through evolution, the knowledge obtained in one organism by using this approach can be readily applied to many organisms. As a component of the overall biofortification research program, nutritional genomics will leverage the massive knowledge base resulting from the enormous investment of the developed world in DNA sequencing of entire organisms plants, bacteria, fungi, and animals. This knowledge base will be used to increase specific micronutrient levels in crops that will be of most benefit to the needs of the developing world. Once the genes of interest are identified, they are moved into a crop species to demonstrate proof of concept to effect the desired change in nutritional content of the target tissues. This process can provide novel traits for breeding that are not available in the existing germplasm betacarotene in rice endosperm, for example. The expanding ability to manipulate pro-vitamin A carotenoid synthesis such as in Golden Rice, vitamin E synthesis, and mineral composition in plants can be directly traced to advancements in nutritional genomics and exemplifies the power and potential benefits of the approach.

Activities to be undertaken in this project area aim to:

- Leverage and integrate new methods in genomics, genetics, and molecular biology to identify and understand plant biosynthetic genes of nutritional importance, specifically those related to zinc, iron, and vitamin A;
- Demonstrate proof of concept nutritional enhancements by engineering genes involved in the

biosynthesis of essential vitamins and accumulation of essential minerals;

- Analyze the consequences of proof of concept enhancements on nutrients and bioavailability;
- Transfer proven materials to partner breeding centers for implementation in Phase 1 and 2 crops;
- Assist with analysis of micronutrient composition and agronomic traits; and
- Aid breeders in identifying molecular markers to nutritionally important genes for incorporation into molecular breeding programs.

On-Farm Testing and Adaptation

The on-farm testing phase is crucial, especially in regions and for crops for which adoption rates of modern varieties have been low. Simply, if the varieties are not grown or appreciated by farmers widely and by large numbers, the positive impacts will not be achieved.

The Scope of Research on Transgenic Crop.

Breeding, dissemination, and impact activities, outlined in the ten-year plan, are focused on development of conventionally-bred crops. No activities involving the release of nutritionally-improved transgenic crops to farmers and consumers are proposed here or are included in proposal budgets for the initial four years for which funding is being requested. Research and development activities with respect to transgenic crops are confined to agricultural research centers and research laboratories. Transgenic methods hold great promise for improving the nutrient content of staple foods and speeding up the breeding process over what can be achieved using conventional methods. High social benefit and lower risk applications, such as the incorporation of desirable traits from crop wild relatives, will be favored throughout the program whenever transgenic methods are considered.

The biofortification challenge program will implement a wide range of technologies including germplasm characterization, breeding, molecular marker assisted breeding and genetic transformation technologies. The mix and extent to which each of these technologies is used will vary by crop see crop appendixes for further information. The first phase of the project will mainly involve germplasm deployment of land races and breeding genotypes. Genetic transformation technologies will be used in the first phase for research purposes to a better understanding of the targeted nutritional pathways resulting in better screening and to develop efficient genomic tools for marker assisted selection and breeding; and in the second and third phases for potential seed deployment by increasing the level of a trait beyond what is available in the gene pool and by providing traits not present in the gene pool.

The project participating institutions have established strict regulations to develop and deploy genetically modified organisms consistent with the CGIAR policy. All institutions involved have well-established guidelines for biosafety related issues and will pursue rigorous scientific processes to ensure the safe use of transgenic plants when there is a high social benefit. Components of the project that involve genetically transformed plants will strictly adhere to international safety standards and the national regulations of the partner countries. As part of their research agenda, several institutions involved in the project are conducting gene flow, risk assessment project and food safety studies. Results from such studies will be incorporated during the implementation of the program.

The Centers will distribute with caution and consultation approval of civil society transgenic materials for experimental purposes with advanced informed consent only to countries where national biosafety legislations are in place.

Development of Golden Rice is much further ahead of any other nutritionally -improved transgenic crop. Research activities related to Golden Rice will be undertaken under the purview of the Biofortification Challenge Program and will adhere to the guidelines set forth above. Research will be undertaken during Phase 1 at IRRI and other collaborating research institutions to evaluate the agronomic and nutritional properties of various existing lines, and to develop experimental lines with even higher levels of beta-carotene. Initial evaluations of the bioavailability of beta-carotene in Golden Rice using human subjects is not expected to be undertaken until 2004. Decisions concerning possible release to farmers and consumers, therefore, can only be taken well after the first four years for which funding is being sought, pending results of an array of agronomic, nutritional, and safety tests.

On-farm research and development remains a program component of many NARS' partners in this proposal and is supported by their collaborating commodity networks (for example, the African bean, cassava, and sweet potato networks). However, staffing and operating costs constraints have been progressively reducing the scale of on-farm research, particularly in some of the key Latin American and African target countries of this biofortification work. While there is a growing body of experience to work with and through these resource constraints, we aim to stimulate further creative on-farm R& D relationships, starting from the strengths of NARS and moving to joint work with, inter alia, civil society groups, farmers' organizations, agricultural schools, and even churches when technically appropriate and mutually beneficial.

Multiplication and Diffusion of Biofortified Varieties

Explicit attention to seed multip lication and diffusion will also be key for the success of the project. Field studies are increasingly showing that certified seed, sold and promoted through formal channels delivers solid results among the more progressive farmers but often bypasses much of the rural poor the cases of Asian rices and African maize hybrids being important exceptions. Hence, a range of channels will be brought into action to ensure that seeds and ultimately the food itself are distributed to the targeted communities where micronutrient deficiencies are widespread. One effective channel used by all of the Future Harvest Centers to distribute improved varieties has been the NARES. In many instances, commodity-based regional research networks also have helped in the exchange and coordination of research, knowledge and germplasm distribution. Action-oriented research has also shown that local and private companies, civil society groups, farmers organizations, women's cooperatives, and specially-formed seed producer groups have proven effective in reaching remote and micro-niche areas, which otherwise might be overlooked by routine seed sector production and diffusion paths. A mix of centralized and decentralized seed production and diffusion arrangements will be supported to ensure a steady supply of the new germplasm, which meets farmer-desired quality standards. Proposal collaborators together have significant and innovative experience to bring to bear here.

Policy Analysis

The CGIAR can be given much of the credit for the fall in staple food prices over the past three decades, which has increased food security among the poor in terms of energy intake. This decline has also freed up resources that would have been spent for food staples. Nonetheless, the growth in supply of some foods, such as pulses, has not kept pace with growth in population and demand, resulting in higher prices for these foods. In the past, economists have most often equated food security with energy security. Consumption of food staples and energy intakes have been the focus of many studies, but relatively little is known about trends in the dietary quality of the poor. Biofortified crops, if successfully developed, can have a large positive impact on micronutrient status. Rigorous cost-effectiveness studies of biofortified crops will need to be undertaken, especially in the context of other food-based interventions. The realized impact of biofortified crops on the micronutrient status of those most deficient in micronutrients will depend on a number of factors:

1. Will there be an income effect in micronutrient-deficient rural areas via improved yields and offfarm linkages? If so, the ability to diversify diets and improve micronutrient status will be enhanced.

2. Will the price of micronutrient-rich foods be reduced for the micronutrient-deficient? This will only happen if market infrastructure is extensive or, when it is not, if farmers in micronutrientdeficient areas can get access to the new seeds.

3. How will rapid urbanization change the demand for biofortified crops and micronutrient-rich foods in general? In terms of the demand for dietary diversity, urbanization can be a positive force for example, through better access to nutrition information and a variety of foods or a negative force such as through greater influence of advertising toward more processed foods that often are expensive sources of micronutrients.

4. How important are non-economic factors in determining consumption of biofortified crops? The organoleptic qualit ies of food are not expected to change dramatically as a result of biofortification. However, the perceptions of the developers of the crop about what is "dramatic" may differ a great deal from the perceptions of the consumer. Even if there is no sensory difference from the consumer's perspective, will there be an effect on consumption simply from knowing that the crop is biofortified?

Partnerships

In simple terms, the biofortification strategy involves adding nutritional quality to an already long list of breeding objectives primarily concerned with improving crop productivity. From this perspective, it is the ultimate responsibility of plant breeders to develop varieties that farmers will want to grow and that have the desired nutritional characteristics. This adaptive breeding work will be carried out primarily by NARES on a country-by-country basis, with assistance from Future Harvest centers in developing breeding tools and in coordinating this work across countries. To be successful, however, this plant breeding work cannot be done in isolation. Plant breeders will need

to pay close attention to human nutritionists for advice on what breeding objectives to pursue levels of nutrients and compounds that inhibit and promote bioavailability and how these are affected by various steps in processing and cooking. Human nutritionists must evaluate the potential of various crop lines to improve nutrition at various points in the breeding process and provide feedback to the breeders. Research in the area of nutritional genomics will provide new ideas for breeding strategies and will make the breeding process more efficient through marker-assisted selection. Use of participatory plant breeding will ensure that, once developed, nutritionally enhanced varieties are acceptable to farmers.

The CGIAR biofortification project has built up strong partnerships to accomplish the basic, applied, and adaptive research and outreach that will be necessary for the adoption of this new technology. A consortium of partner organizations and institutions brought into the project through competitive bidding will undertake the individual components of project activities as described below. Each member of the project team has been selected based on their unique comparative advantage to contribute to the goals of the project.

2

Zinc adds "Micro-Power" to Crop Nutrition

Zinc is as essential for plant growth as is nitrogen (N), phosphorus (P) or any of the other 16 essential elements. The micro amounts of zinc required for plant growth are related to the type of work it performs. Like potassium (K) it is heavily involved in enzyme activation which serves to regulate plant growth activity. A shortage of zinc is most often noted when plants are in an early stage of growth. Thus, zinc is closely associated with both phosphorus (P) and nitrogen (N) performance. Research helps to document how zinc nutrition management practices contribute to improved crop growth and profitability.

When do high yielding crops need zinc

A 180 bushel corn crop must absorb nearly one half pound of zinc during the growing season. It is not uncommon for growers to apply 5-8 pounds of zinc to get a more uniform distribution of zinc. Zinc must be available for use throughout the growing season so a 100% water soluble product is not always the best choice. Peak zinc needs differ with the crop and responsiveness to zinc applications vary as shown in the table. Corn shows leaf chlorosis and stunted plants during the first few weeks. A shortage appears later with beans as flower buds shed or with cotton as growth and fruiting are delayed. Thus, most crops need a readily available supply of zinc for both early and late season growth and yield development.

Importance of balanced nutrition

Proper nitrogen management has received the most attention in crop nutrition, but it should be noted that micronutrients such as zinc are important in getting the most out of an investment in NPK fertilizer. Zinc is heavily involved in enzyme functions essential for regulating plant growth. Zinc, nitrogen and phosphorus are essential for rapid stem and leaf formation, for seed development and for other vital growth activities that create crop yield and quality. As tillage is reduced and surface crop residues increase, seedbeds remain cool and moist. These conditions tend to slow zinc and phosphorus uptake by a smaller root system.

Impact of zinc levels on yield

High crop yields are not possible without zinc, even though it is needed in very small amounts. Soils might contain anywhere from a few to several hundred pounds of zinc. Fine textured soils often contain more zinc than coarse textured soils. University of Georgia soils lab has established 2 lbs/a as a low testing soil and 2-8 lbs as a medium soil test range. Such low levels of availability have been reported across the country and crop responses have been measured. Kansas research showed that rates of 0, 2, and 4 pounds of zinc per acre increased soybean yields from 30 to 46 and 50 bu/a, respectively. The zinc leaf composition increased from 18 to 25 and 29 ppm as the yield increased. Kentucky studies revealed that a row application was the most consistent method for applying zinc to responsive soils.

Soil pH zinc availability declines as soil pH increases. Crop response to Zn increases as soil pH increases from 6 to 7 or higher.

Soil texture fine textured soils are less responsive than coarse textured soils due in part to a higher cation exchange capacity and a larger reservoir of zinc and other nutrients.

Soil phosphorus level coarse textured soils testing medium to low in zinc and high in phosphorus are most likely to respond to fertilizer zinc.

Organic matter zinc is closely associated with the organic fraction of soil. As microorganisms decompose residues, zinc becomes available.

Subsoil zinc the subsoil is a poor provider of zinc since zinc moves little in the soil, plant root growth is limited and organic matter is low.

Reduced tillage zinc absorption by seedling plants is difficult when soils are cold and wet and plant roots are growing at a slow pace.

Of these factors, five are directly related to soil conditions. In promoting agricultural productivity, it is essential that the role of soil be acknowledged and its important functions be valued and protected. Both crop productivity and harvest quality are clearly influenced by having the correct balance of essential nutrients present in the soil. Scientific trials going back for hundreds of years have repeatedly demonstrated that when any plant nutrient is lacking, crop growth and quality will be adversely impacted. When fertilizers are properly used in combination with locally available manures or cover crops, nutrient deficiencies and imbalances are corrected. Fertilizers come from natural products and contain the essential nutrients for the growth of healthy plants plants that are used directly for human consumption, feed for animals, supplying fiber, producing biofuels, or growing timber. Human and animal survival depends on the growth of healthy plants.

Fertilizers are currently used in two ways:

(1) To improve unfavorable conditions for plant growth by overcoming pre-existing deficiencies commonly called build up of soil fertility reserves.

(2) To replace the quantity of nutrients removed in crop

harvest commonly called maintenance of soil fertility reserves.

As an example, where soil improvement through phosphorus (P) fertilization has been practiced for a number of years, it may not be necessary to apply more nutrient than is removed in the harvested crop. However, in many soils of the world, it is still necessary to build and improve their nutrient status so they can reach their potential to support healthy plant growth. In such conditions, additions larger than crop removal are required to build the nutrient reservoir in the soil. Soil testing is essential for knowing what scenario is most appropriate for each specific field.

In many regions, we observe that high levels of N fertilization without appropriate inputs of other essential nutrients have a negative effect on both crop production and the environment. Nitrogen fertilization where P or K are lacking typically results in enhanced nitrate leaching losses and denitrification. Crops without balanced nutrition may suffer from excessive lodging, unfavorable weed and pest competition, lower yields, and reduced harvest quality. Much of the early research on crop nutrition focused on the plant's need for each single nutrient. Although modern research is more complicated, we now recognize that more emphasis should be given to the interactions between nutrients. Ensuring the efficient use of plant nutrients requires that all essential elements are present at the optimal concentration to meet times of peak nutrient demand.

Balanced crop nutrition requires the proper supply of N, P, and K plus other nutrients such as magnesium, calcium, sulfur, and micronutrients as determined by soil and crop analysis.

There are very few "ideal" soils in the world; that is, soils that contain all of the essential nutrients in the proper balance required by crops. Overcoming these pre-existing deficiencies is the goal of the fertilizer industry. Animal manures are excellent at providing many of the essential nutrients for crops, but their composition is rarely in balance with what the soil requires to adequately supply the plant's needs. Similarly, legume cover crops are especially good as a N source for subsequent crops; but provide no other additional nutrients that were not already in the soil. The concept of balanced plant nutrition is certainly not a new one, but it is still not adequately understood and practiced. It is time to move beyond the concept of managing single nutrients.

Understanding pH management and plant nutrition

A wide range of substrates are available on the market to grow orchids, or many other plants. Some people are using substrates manufactured by large companies for the production of container grown crops other than orchids. Other people are using substrates manufactured primarily for growing orchids. Still others are blending their own substrates from individual components.

The choice of substrates will affect the effectiveness of your fertilizer program. Substrates can differ substantially in both their physical properties and chemical properties. In part 4 or this series, we will discuss key aspects of physical and chemical properties, and also leaching, and how these factors affect plant nutrition.

Physical properties

Physical properties deal with the ratio of air water solid in a substrate. Container substrates should be thought of as a sponge. A sponge is made up of the material used to make the sponge solid space and holes pore spaces. If a material has a high bulk density high weight per unit volume, then a sponge of this material would have a lot of solid space with little pore space. Examples of high bulk density materials are sand, clays, or field soils. In comparison, a sponge made from materials that have a low bulk density (low weight per unit volume) would have little solid space but lots of pore spaces. Examples of low bulk density materials are peat, coir, bark, vermiculite, things commonly found in container substrates.

Pore space can be filled with either air or water. The ratio of air to water in a given substrate will depend on size and distribution of the pores. During an irrigation, small pores called micropores tend to fill completely with water, while large pores called macropores tend to drain, which allows air to get back into the substrate. It has been said that after an irrigation, the ideal container substrate would have 25% of its volume taken up with pores filled with air, 60% of its volume taken up with pores filled with water, and the remaining 15% taken up with solids.

To put numbers on these values, an "average" 6 inch (15-cm) azalea pot has a volume of about 1.6 liters. The volume of air, water, and solid occupied by the "ideal" substrate in this pot would be 0.4 liters of air space, 0.96 liters of water, and 0.24 liters of solid. In general, substrates used for propagation tend to be very fine lots of micropores and so hold more water on a relative basis at the expense of air space when compared to the "ideal" substrate. Coarse substrates have lots of macropores and so have greater air space at the expense of water.

Container height also affects the ratio of air:water held in a substrate after an irrigation. In general, the shorter the height of the container, the greater the percentage of pore space that is filled with water and the lower the air space. For example, after a thorough watering, the average air and water porosity of five different commercially available root media in a 6 inch (15 cm) tall pot was 19% (air) and 64% (water), in a 4 inch (10 cm) tall pot was 13% (air) and 70% (water), in a 3 inch (8 cm) tall cell bedding flat was 7% (air) and 76% (water), and a 1 inch (2.5 cm) tall plug flat was 2% (air) and 82% (water), respectively. The percentage of solid material in the root media remained constant in the different container sizes. It was the ratio of air space to water space that changed with the different container heights. This is one reason why it is easier to overwater a small pot than it is a large pot because the air space in the small pot is lower than that found in the larger pot after an irrigation.

Finally, the ability of a substrate to absorb water will affect physical properties. Ideal physical properties are measured in a laboratory by allowing the substrate to remain submersed in water for 24 hours before allowing it to drain (the difference between the saturated weight and drained weight (in grams) is a measure of air porosity). In comparison, a typically irrigation may last for only 30 seconds or less. That means that under a typical irrigation, most substrates will not rewet to maximum saturation, resulting in more air space and less water-holding capacity than is measured in a laboratory test.

Another problem with organic substrates like peat and (especially) bark, is that they become waterrepellent if allowed to dry too much. Commercial substrates will often contain a wetting agent or surfactant that aids in rewetting (increases water absorption). For long-term greenhouse crops, like hanging baskets, it is often recommended to reapply a surfactant to the substrate every month or two because Not for publication or reproduction without the authors consent.

Chemical properties

Chemical properties generally refer to a substrates ability to buffer the water held in the substrate against changes in either pH or nutrition. The term most often used to describe chemical properties is cation exchange capacity or CEC. CEC refers to the ability of substrate particles (such as peat) to absorb and release positively charged cations like potassium, ammonium, calcium, or magnesium, thus buffering the substrate against sudden changes in pH or nutrient levels.

An example of how CEC affects pH and nutrient management occurs when a fertilizer solution is applied to a substrate. A fertilizer high in ammoniacal-nitrogen produces acid (H+). The acid is absorbed by the substrate and a different cation, usually calcium, is released. Conversely, a fertilizer high in nitratenitrogen usually calcium nitrate based produces base. The base causes an acid (H+) bound by the substrate to be released, which will then react with the base to produce water or CO2. In both cases, the net result is that the pH and calcium concentrations remain stable. Substrates that have high CEC (more buffered) can resist a change in pH for long periods of time, whereas pH can change very rapidly in substrates that have low CEC (less buffered). CEC can play an important role in pH buffering when a field soil is added to a container substrate. CEC-based pH and nutrient buffering does occur with field soils because the substrate has a high bulk density (weight). In contrast to field soils, research has shown that the CEC of peat, coir, or bark-based substrates has little effect on resisting change in pH or in supplying nutrients.

This does not mean that the substrate plays no role in pH or nutritional management. Peat tends to be very acidic. Limestone is commonly added to peatbased substrates to neutralize the acidity and bring the pH up to an acceptable level for plant growth. The amount of acidity found in most acidic peats will not be neutralized very quickly by bases found in irrigation water. Using the example given in Part 2 of this series, a limestone incorporation rate of 5 pounds per cubic yard will supply approximately 100 meq of limestone per 6 inch (15-cm) pot. Applying 16 fluid ounces (0.5 liters) of water containing 250 ppm alkalinity to that 6 inch pot will supply about 2.5 meq of lime. That means that 40 irrigations are required to equal the amount of base found in 5 pounds of limestone. If you are only watering once a week, then it will take 40 weeks to bring the substrate pH up to an acceptable level. If you are using a pure water source without any alkalinity, then you may never get the pH up to an acceptable level. The presence of limestone in the substrate has also been shown to increase the buffering capacity when using acidic fertilizer solutions.

Finally, substrate degradation will affect nutrition and pH management. Degradation is the breakdown of the substrate, similar to composting. Of all the materials commonly found in container substrates, bark is the least stable, and therefore the most susceptible to degradation. The problem with degradation is that it not only absorbs all the nitrogen present (causing nitrogen starvation), but the process also tends to be very acidic. Hardwood barks tend to be the most stable. Softwood barks usually require some composting to make them stable. If a bark (any bark) contains any wood, then it is unacceptable for use in container substrates because the wood will cause will cause rapid degradation and nitrogen absorption.

Leaching

Leaching is the application of water or fertilizer solution beyond what can be held by the substrate. Applying extra water is recommended to thoroughly wet the substrate, and to remove excess salts from the substrate. The leaching fraction is the volume of water that drains from the substrate relative to the volume of water applied. For example, if you apply 15 fluid ounces (0.44 liters) of water, and 3 fluid ounces (0.08 liters) comes out of the bottom of the pot then 3 divided by 15, then times 100 equals a 20% leaching fraction. In other words, 20% of the water applied to the plant came out of the bottom of the pot.

It is generally taught that you should have between a 10% and 20% leaching fraction with every watering. However, research has shown that leaching is not necessary for long periods of time if you have a good water source (RO or rain water is ideal) and the fertilizer you use does not contain any harmful salts like sodium or chloride. There are reasons to leach pots, usually because the fertilizer concentration that is applied to the crop is too high for the growth rate, or the water quality is poor, and unused salts (like calcium, magnesium, or sodium) build up in the substrate. In general, whether or not you leach should be based on soil test information showing salt levels actually building up in the substrate, rather than because somebody tells you too.

Leaching rates also affect the optimal fertilizer concentration for your crop. Research has shown that the same nutrient levels could be maintained in a peat based substrate if a solution containing 400 ppm nitrogen were applied with 50% leaching or a solution containing 100 ppm nitrogen were applied with

0% leaching. This research also showed that applying a solution containing 400 ppm nitrogen with 0% leaching rapidly lead to salts building up in the substrate to unacceptable levels, while applying a solution containing 100 ppm nitrogen with 50% leaching lead to nutrient deficiencies because there wasn't enough of the fertilizer remaining in the pot because of the excess leaching.

Applying fertilizer to a substrate

When you apply fertilizer to a substrate, which is more important, the concentration of the fertilizer solution, or the volume that you apply? In fact, both are important because as a plant grows, it adds mass, and a portion of this mass is made up of fertilizer nutrients. It has been shown in a number of experiments that it is the amount of fertilizer applied to a crop that affects crop quality, not simply the fertilizer concentration.

To calculate the amount of fertilizer applied, you need to know both the fertilizer concentration and the volume applied. For example, applying 1 liter (about 1 quart) of a fertilizer solution containing 100 ppm (100 mg nitrogen/liter) will supply 100 mg of nitrogen. If only 0.5 liters (about 1 pint) were applied of the same fertilizer solution, then only 50 mg of nitrogen would be applied.

This can be especially important when you are only applying fertilizer on a weekly basis. If the amount of fertilizer solution being absorbed into the substrate decreases for any reason (decreased waterholding capacity), they you could end up starving your plants.

How do commercial growers manage pH and nutrient levels

Commercial growers have learned that a single fertilizer concentration may or may not work depending on a number of factors including leaching, growth rates, light levels, irrigation frequency, etc. Instead, many growers will manage the pH or nutrient level within the substrate itself. This requires that the grower tests the pH, electrical conductivity, and perhaps even the specific nutrient levels contained in the substrate on a regular basis. These measured values can be used to make adjustments to the fertilizer solution. For example, if the substrate pH is too high, then a grower might switch to a fertilizer containing more ammoniacal nitrogen, or they may lower the alkalinity of the water. If the EC of the substrate is too high, the grower may increase the leaching rate, or decrease the concentration of fertilizer applied to the crop. The point is that by measuring the pH and EC of the substrate, they can make sure that a particular fertilizer solution is doing what they think it is doing, and make changes if things are going wrong, usually long before there are noticeable problems with the plant.

Even though there is not a lot of specific knowledge about acceptable ranges for substrate pH and EC with orchids, it is probable that they are similar to almost all other crops and so will grow best in a substrate pH around 6.0. Because they appear to be somewhat salt sensitive, they will also grow best with a substrate EC slightly lower than the optimal level recommended for most crops. If testing with a pourthru method, then the desired substrate EC would be between 1 and 2 mS/cm.

Monitoring Media pH and Nutrient Levels

For successful pH and nutritional management of container grown crops, the goal is to keep the pH and nutritional levels within an acceptable range and to spot problem trends early on. This is a far better strategy than blindly applying fertilizer and hoping everything is OK, or having to take dramatic steps to rescue stressed plants. Using reliable meters, you can measure pH and electrical conductivity or EC in substrates. Other advantages or in-house testing are that the tests are inexpensive and the results to be obtained quickly, typically in less than 1or 2 hours. How often do you test? Typically commercial growers will test substrate pH and EC every 2 to 3 weeks. That does not mean they test every pot or every crop every two or three weeks.

Instead, they may do some random sampling to make sure everything is pH and EC are within acceptable levels, or they may test a few know problem crops and then assume that if their pH and EC are within acceptable levels, then other, less sensitive crops are not having problems. There are a number of different testing methods commonly used for measuring the pH and EC in container substrates.

Step 1. Collect a small amount of substrate from the bottom 2/3rd of the pot. For very small plants, like those being grown in plug trays or bedding flats, use the whole cell as a sample. Take samples from 5 to 10 or more plants distributed in the group of plants to be sampled. When a sufficient amount of substrate is collected, thoroughly mix the sample to ensure uniformity.

Step 2. Measure out a known volume of substrate in a beaker or cup [usually 2-4 oz. (50 to 100 ml)]. The beaker should be firmly filled with the substrate so that it is slightly more compressed than when it was in the pot. Place 2 equal volume of distilled water into cup. Allow the solution to equilibrate (30-60 minutes) before measuring pH and EC.

Step 3. Measure pH and EC directly in the slurry.

Step 1. Collect a small amount of substrate from the bottom 2/3rd of the pot. For very small plants, like those being grown in plug trays or bedding flats, use the whole cell as a sample. Take samples from 5 to 10 or more plants distributed in the group of plants to be sampled. When a sufficient amount of substrate is collected, thoroughly mix the sample to ensure uniformity.

Step 2. About 4 to 8 oz (150 to 300 ml) of fresh substrate is placed in a cup. Distilled water is slowly added while the sample is constantly stirred with a spatula or knife until it has reached a consistent moisture level. This is determined to be when the sample behaves like a paste, the surface glistens with water, but there is no free water on the surface of the sample. The solution is allowed to equilibrate for 60 minutes

Step 3. Measure pH directly in the slurry.

Step 4. Extract the solution from the media by squeezing slurry through paper towel or a coffee filter. Measure EC in extracted solution.

Step 1. Irrigate the crop one hour before testing, making sure the substrate is thoroughly wet. Allow the pots to drain for 30-60 minutes.

Step 2. Once drainage has stopped, place the pot to be sampled into a plastic saucer and pour onto the surface enough distilled water to get about 2 oz. (50 ml) to come out of the bottom of the pot.

Step 3. Measure pH and EC directly in the leachate

Step 1. Irrigate the crop one hour before testing, making sure the substrate is thoroughly wet. Allow the pots to drain for 30-60 minutes.

Step 2. Collect a small amount of substrate from the bottom 2/3rd of the pot. For very small plants, like those being grown in plug trays or bedding flats, use the whole cell as a sample. Take samples from 5 to 10 or more plants distributed in the group of plants to be sampled. When a sufficient amount of substrate is collected, thoroughly mix the sample to ensure uniformity.

Step 3. Squeeze the solution from the media. For a cleaner sample, media can be squeezed through a paper towel or coffee filter. The volume of solution needed will depend on the type of pH or EC meter used for testing.

Step 4. Measure the pH and EC in the extracted solution

In general, there is no one "best" method for measuring substrate-pH or EC in the greenhouse. However, with orchids, especially with specimen plants, the pour-thru method may work best because it will not damage roots. Other reasons for deciding on which method to use in your greenhouse include any experience that you have with a particular method as well as how much help and advice you can get from other people that are close by such as other growers, extension agents, universities, or soil testing laboratories.

Whichever soil testing method you choose, consistency is the key to making that method work. Consistency starts with having a single, trained person taking the test.

Other tips include:

(1) Choose one soil testing method and stick with it. Different methods can give different results.

(2) When removing substrate from the pot, take the sample from the bottom 2/3rd of the pot. The bottom 2/3rd is typically were the roots are in the pot and sampling in this way avoids fertilizer salts that can accumulate at the substrate surface with all irrigation methods (not just subirrigation).

(3) Try to take media samples roughly the same time before or after an irrigation. This is especially important with the squeeze method.

4) Choose a reliable pH and EC meter and calibrate it regularly. Calibrating solution has an expiration day and should be discarded when that date is reached.

An understanding of these links offers guidance on nutrition-relevant actions that provide sustainable solutions to environmental changes. At a time of unprecedented climatic and environmental change, nutrition knowledge becomes vital in enabling individuals and populations to adapt in the most positive manner possible.The nutritional status of populations, as a recognizable and measurable outcome, should help direct other scientific disciplines and intervention programs in identifying sustainable solutions to the environmental and economic problems facing global communities.

The Environment-Nutrition Connection

As community development priorities merge with those

of environmental conservation, it becomes increasingly clear that unless human populations meet their basic survival needs they cannot afford to conserve. At the same time unless local communities protect the environments around them they have limited hope to thrive beyond the short term. As nutrition represents the most fundamental of human needs, it provides a useful perspective from which to address this paradox. Nutrition research provides essential information on how environmental degradation can lead to major nutrition-related health problems such as malnutrition, infectious disease, and contamination.When people have reduced access to and intake of crucial bioresources, they may suffer from protein-energy

Nutrition and The Environment

Environmental contamination from industrial and agricultural chemicals such as heavy metals,organochlorines, and radionucleotides may compromise people's nutritional status and health either directly or through changes in diet.

Some research and intervention programs have focused on providing micronutrients such as vitamin A or minerals through genetic improvement, crop diversification, and soil management. More attention needs to be applied,however, to identifying crop varieties and minor crops with selective nutritional assets such as micronutrients, soluble fiber, or antioxidants and to analyzing the nutritional content of indigenous fruits and vegetables and wild edible species.Programs should give greater importance to maintaining the genetic diversity of plant species within home gardens and local agroecosystems. Where they can be exploited sustainably, uncultivated resources can also improve nutrition indirectly by contributing to economic livelihood.

Genetic modification and other strategies that target single nutrients promise selective improvement of plant nutrient composition. Although genetically modified organisms are subject to considerable scrutiny for their potential adverse effects on human health, this technology also has potential ecological and social effects that require careful evaluation.

While institutional approaches are essential to address problems of a global magnitude,national efforts, particularly those involving local communities, are also important. Local multidisciplinary activities that combine nutrition research, ethnobotany, and ecosystem and resource management with health care activities, and that embrace participatory models of empowerment and initiative,offer real hope for addressing problems at the levels where people are directly affected.

Traditional values of conservation, encompassing relationships to land,' spiritual dimensions, and concepts of health, are fragile and vulnerable to modern forces of change. Nonetheless, cultural values can be important components in programs of public health education and ecological recovery. Integrating the biological, social, and cultural dimensions of human-environmental relations is as essential to the present and future sustainability of human health as it has been throughout history.

Conclusion

Major health problems of the 21st century include nutritional deficiencies and dietary changes in both rural and urban settings. Nutritional analyses, combined with an understanding of traditional systems and resources, can help identify the biological and sociocultural components of solutions to dietary and health problems associated with dietary change and adaptive strategies for the future.Addressing nutritional needs offers a primary rationale for the preservation of traditional knowledge and life-styles, the conservation of wild and cultivated resources, and the sustainable use of the environments in which they are located.

3

Guide to Efficient Plant Nutrition Management

Plant nutrients are essential for producing sufficient and healthy food for the world's expanding population. Plant nutrients are therefore a vital component of any system of sustainable agriculture. Moreover, agricultural intensification requires increased flows of plant nutrients to crops and higher uptake of those nutrients by crops. The depletion of nutrient stocks in the soil, which is occurring in many developing countries, is a major but often hidden form of land degradation. On the other hand, excessive applications of nutrients, or inefficient management, can cause environmental problems, especially if large quantities of nutrients are lost from the soil/ crop system into water or the air. The *Guide to efficient plant nutrition management* addresses some major issues related to the agronomic management of plant nutrients in an attempt to ensure both enhanced and sustainable agricultural production and to safeguard the environment.

This guide is intended to promote the assessment of plant nutrient requirements on a farming system basis and monitoring of soil fertility. It will help in the formulation of advice to governments and eventually legislation in the field of fertilizer use and plant nutrition. As the guide emphasizes, plant nutrient management should be a major concern at both the farmer and the national level.

The guide is intended to assist everyone concerned with the manufacture, marketing and use of fertilizers in working towards efficient and sustainable plant nutrition management. The advice it contains should be promoted by governments in regional groupings, by international and national non-governmental organizations, by the fertilizer industry and by United Nations agencies.

All parties addressed by this guide are invited to observe and promote its general principles. The cooperation of the fertilizer industry in observing these principles will be particularly valuable. As a follow-up, soil fertility status and the evolution of soil fertility should be evaluated and monitored by agro-ecological zone. Particular emphasis should be put on long-term trends in soil fertility so that plant nutrient depletion, wherever observed, can be countered. Environmental impact assessments should be carried out regularly, especially in zones with intensive use of fertilizers.

The challenges for plant nutrition management are to maintain and where possible increase sustainable crop productivity to meet demands for food and raw materials, and to enhance the quality of land and water resources. There is no contradiction between these challenges. Indeed, environmental hazards can be minimized by matching plant nutrients with crop requirements, and judicious soil and water conservation methods. Agriculture inevitably removes plant nutrients from the soil and from the farm. Consequently, if a farming system is to be sustainable, these nutrients have to be replaced by whatever sources are available. For the farmer, nutrient losses are money wasted. In many developing countries, the loss of soil fertility from continual nutrient mining by crop removal without adequate replenishment, combined with imbalanced plant nutrition practices, poses a serious threat to agricultural production. It is already causing yield decreases as large as those caused by other forms of environmental degradation.

While recycling and transfer of nutrients from noncrop areas, crop residues and animal manure can partially make up for exports of nutrients by harvested products, the use of external sources such as mineral fertilizers is essential to meet crop requirements and to increase crop production in many farming systems. Intensification of agriculture by increasing the use of plant nutrients is limited by environmental hazards and economic constraints. In industrialized countries, environmental issues and international trade agreements restricting surplus food production are now the limiting factors on further intensification; in developing countries, the high cost of external sources of nutrients and their inadequate availability limit intensification.

Challenges for plant nutrition management

The objectives are to set forth responsibilities and propose guidelines for all parties engaged in or influencing the production, distribution and use of plant nutrients, with special reference to fertilizers.

Reference is made to the shared responsibility of many segments of society, including governments, individually or in regional groupings, industry, trade, international institutions and farmers, to work together with a common aim: an efficient use of plant nutrients that will lead to intensified and sustainable agriculture and protection of the natural resource base. The guide specifically aims to:

- Promote a better understanding of the role of plant nutrients in securing the sustainability of agriculture and in building up and maintaining soil productivity;

- Ensure that all sources of plant nutrients, especially fertilizers, are used efficiently for increased agricultural production;
- Identify how the application of plant nutrients can affect the environment and point to ways of avoiding negative impacts;
- Formulate recommendations for plant nutrition management in a framework of IPNS, taking into account farmers' production goals and strategies within specific agroecological, social and economic conditions;
- Promote the development of sound advisory services and efficient input supply systems to farmers;
- Facilitate the emergence of farmers' associations leading to the adoption of sound plant nutrition practices; and
- Provide elements for the design of national strategies and policies for effective plant nutrition in support of agricultural intensification and rural development.

The answer depends on the ecological, social and economic characteristics of each farming system. Increased attention is now being paid to developing Integrated Plant Nutrition Systems that maintain or enhance soil productivity through a balanced use of mineral fertilizers combined with organic sources of plant nutrients, including biological nitrogen fixation. IPNS is ecologically, socially and economically viable, and it can increase both soil productivity and crop yields. It focuses first on the seasonal or annual cropping system, rather than on an individual crop; secondly, on the management of plant nutrients in the whole farming system; and, thirdly, on the concept of village or community areas rather than individual fields. The FAO study *World agriculture: towards 2010* estimates that about two-thirds of the needed increase in crop production in developing countries will have to come from yield increases on land already under cultivation.

Plant nutrients are the most important inputs for increasing yields. Over the past three decades, additional nutrients applied as fertilizer have been responsible for 55 percent of the yield increases in developing countries. The development of plant nutrition management to increase the quantity of plant nutrients in farming systems and thus crop productivity is a major challenge for food security and rural development.

This guide promotes the effective management of plant nutrients. It is relevant to farmers, advisory services, research and extension bodies, development agencies, financial institutions, the fertilizer industry and government decision-makers in both developed and developing countries in fact to all those concerned with sustainable agricultural production and environmental protection.

Nature and supply of plant nutrients

Plants build up their biomass using water, carbon dioxide from the air, energy from sunlight and nutrients taken up from the soil and water. For optimum plant growth, nutrients must be available:

- as solutes in the soil water;
- in adequate and balanced amounts, corresponding to the instant demand of the crop;
- in a form which is accessible to the root system (except when provided through foliage).

Plants are supplied with nutrients mainly from:

- soil reserves;
- mineral fertilizers;
- organic sources;
- atmospheric nitrogen through biological fixation;

- aerial deposition caused by wind and rain;
- irrigation, flood or groundwater, and sedimentation from runoff.

These sources are used by farmers according to their availability and affordability. The total amount of plant nutrients available to the crop is a key factor determining yield.

Plant nutrients

These are elements that are essential for plant growth and that are taken up from the soil or from water irrigation, flood or groundwater or are supplied via a hydroponic medium. The primary nutrients are nitrogen, phosphorus and potassium which are consumed in relatively large amounts. Three secondary nutrients are taken up in smaller quantities but are essential for plant growth: calcium, magnesium and sulphur. Micronutrients or trace elements are required in very small quantities but are often important for plant or animal metabolism. They include iron, zinc, manganese, boron, copper, molybdenum and chlorine. In addition, some plants benefit from the presence of sodium, cobalt and silicon but these do not rank as essential nutrients.

Soil reserves

Soils contain natural reserves of plant nutrients in quantities that depend on soil composition and stage of weathering. These reserves are often in forms unavailable to plants, and only a minor portion is released each year through biological activity or chemical processes. This release is too slow to compensate for the removal of nutrients from agricultural production, especially in the humid tropics where soils are strongly weathered. The quantities of plant nutrients available for a crop are determined by the supply of nutrients to the crop from internal and external sources, the uptake of nutrients by the crop, and losses of plant nutrient to the environment. Thus plant nutrient stock is constantly changing. The capacity of a soil to store easily-available plant nutrients is an important factor in plant nutrition management. Chemical analysis can provide an approximation of the nutrient stock, the accuracy of which is related to soil type, cropping conditions and crop species.

Fertilizers

These are mineral or organic substances, natural or manufactured, that are applied to soil, irrigation water or a hydroponic medium, to supply plants with nutrients. Fertilizers contain at least 5 percent of one or more of the three primary nutrients. The term is often used as an abbreviation for mineral fertilizers. Products with less than 5 percent of combined plant nutrients are called plant nutrient sources. The legal definition of a fertilizer varies in different countries.

Sources of plant nutrients

Mineral fertilizers

Mineral fertilizers are manufactured in liquid or solid form, usually in an industrial process. They can supply main nutrients, secondary nutrients, micronutrients or mixtures of nutrients. Straight fertilizers supply only one nutrient while complex fertilizers supply several. Compound fertilizers are produced by the blending or chemical linkage of straight fertilizers or nutrients. The terms chemical or artificial fertilizers are often used for these products but are misleading because the nutrients supplied by mineral fertilizers are the same as those supplied by the mineralization of organic material through soil micro-organisms; indeed, some fertilizers are directly derived from natural products such as guano, potassium salts or natural sodium nitrates.

Mineral fertilizers have a higher plant nutrient content and a lower bulk than organic sources of plant nutrients. High-grade fertilizers contain more plant nutrients (up to 82 percent) than low-grade fertilizers, producing savings on transport and handling costs.

Organic sources

These nutrients are materials of organic origin, either

natural or processed. The term organic fertilizers is often used incorrectly to describe nutrient sources containing less than 5 percent of at least one of the three primary nutrients. In this sense, some organic materials of animal origin such as guano, bone meal, fishmeal, and blood are true fertilizers but commonly used organic sources of nutrients, such as manure, slurry, compost and sewage sludge, are not. Organic materials can be used to increase the amount of organic matter in the soil, thus enhancing its water retention and exchange capacity, and its physical condition.

Farmyard or animal manure is a mixture of animal excreta and the litter used for bedding. Green manure is fresh, locally produced plant material that is worked into the soil without composting or digestion by animals. When leguminous crops are used as green manure, the atmospheric nitrogen they have fixed is also added to the soil. Slurry is a mixture of liquid and solid animal excreta, sometimes diluted with water. Sludge is residual organic material derived from sewage. Compost consists of organic materials of animal and plant origin partially decomposed through fermentation; mineral fertilizers are sometimes added to it.

Biological nitrogen fixation

Some micro-organisms are able to convert nitrogen in the air to ammonia for use as their nitrogen source. The conversion is made by bacteria living either on their own in the soil or, on a considerably larger scale, in symbiosis with leguminous plants or trees (*rhizobium*), or other specific trees (*actinomycetes*), or with azolla in aquatic conditions. Biological nitrogen fixation can be enhanced by inoculation with efficient strains of nitrogen-fixing micro-organisms, part of the fixed nitrogen being directly assimilated by plants. The term biofertilizers is sometimes inappropriately used for these micro-organisms; microbial inoculants is the preferred term.

Aerial deposition

Some nutrients are supplied in small quantities to the soil surface through aerial deposition. These include nitrates in rainwater, ammonia as a gas or dissolved in rainwater, sulphur in acid rain, salts and chlorine in marine spray and calcium in the form of dust.

Irrigation water, floodwater and groundwater

These sources also supply plant nutrients, either naturally or because fertilizers have been added to the irrigation water. While water often contains small amounts of nutrients, irrigation can also result in a loss of nutrients from leaching. Some of the nutrients provided by surface and groundwater originate from plant nutrient losses within the watershed.

Soil amendments

Amendments are substances that are applied to the soil to correct a major constraint other than low nutrient content. Lime, for example, is used to remedy acidity; phosphates are used to reduce phosphorus fixation; gypsum is used to improve sodic (alkali) soils; and peat can be added to the surface layers to increase organic matter content.

Gathering sources of plant nutrients

The natural plant nutrients found in the soil are deposited there either from the air or from water, or result from nitrogen fixation and the weathering of mineral particles in the soil. Vegetation takes up some of these nutrients, some are geographically redistributed by runoff, and some are lost by volatilization, fixation and leaching. Farmers harvest the natural supply of these nutrients for their crops and reorganize their distribution in space and time through their production systems.

On land under natural vegetation, the organic matter that accumulates at the soil surface releases plant nutrients as it decomposes (or when it is burnt in a fire). Nutrients taken up from deeper layers thus eventually become available to plants in the topsoil. Slashand- burn systems exploit this nutrient management technique. As crops are harvested, the local supply of nutrients is progressively depleted; eventually the land must be left in a prolonged fallow or replenished with external nutrients.

The practice of allowing short fallow periods on arable land is another means of accumulating the natural supply of nutrients for a later cropping period. However, much less nutrients are gathered in a short fallow period than in a long fallow, of ten years or more, in perennial vegetation.

Farming systems redistribute and concentrate natural nutrients in a number of ways. For example:

- some traditional farming systems allow livestock to graze a large non-cropped area and the manure is then collected and spread over a selected cropped area;
- forest litter is collected and used to mulch a cropped area;
- manure from animals kept in corrals and shelters is spread on cropped areas;
- feedstuffs are imported to the farm and fed to livestock whose manure is then spread over cropped areas;
- crop residues are collected and processed (by composting or in biogas plants) and then spread on cropped areas; and
- leguminous crops are grown to supply the plant nutrients that are produced by nitrogen fixation.

Restoring, maintaining and increasing soil fertility are major agricultural priorities, particularly in the many parts of the developing world where soils are inherently poor in plant nutrients, and the demand for food and raw materials is increasing rapidly. In these areas, there is a need to intensify crop production to meet demand for food without using former land fallow practices. A fertile soil provides a sound basis for flexible food production systems that, within the constraints of soil and climate, can grow a wide range of crops to meet changing needs.

Integrated Plant Nutrition Systems

IPNS associate available, accessible and affordable plant nutrients to increase farm productivity and economic returns.

IPNS operate at plot, farm and village or territory levels. At the plot level, they are designed to optimize the uptake of plant nutrients by the crop and increase the productivity of that uptake (the ratio between harvested products and nutrient uptake) while reducing nutrient losses. The optimal nutrient supply is determined by the production methods used, the prevailing prices of fertilizers, the cost of mobilizing local nutrient sources and the commercial value of the crop. IPNS increases plant nutrient stocks in soils and improves other aspects of soil fertility such as water infiltration and water-holding capacity; it also reduces limitations on crop growth caused by factors such as soil acidity and compaction. IPNS make use of crop rotations to optimize nitrogen fixation, the efficient management of crop residues, exploration of the soil by developing rooting systems, and management methods that limit nutrient losses (by exploiting nutrients that are released slowly from organic and mineral sources).

At farm level, IPNS aim to optimize the productivity of the flows of nutrients passing through the farming system during a crop rotation. IPNS improve the production capacity of farmers through application of external plant nutrient sources and amendments, efficient processing, and recycling of crop residues and on-farm organic wastes that limit plant nutrient losses. IPNS empower farmers by increasing their technical know-how and decision-making capacity, and promote changes in land use, crop rotations, and interactions among forestry, livestock and cropping systems in support of agricultural intensification.

IPNS require financial and labour investments, generate additional income and promote an increased rate of return from all inputs. IPNS involve risk management and enhance the synergy among crop, water and plant nutrition management. At the level of the village or farming community,

IPNS take into account plant nutrient sources outside the cropped areas. These include plant nutrients in irrigation water and flood sediments, manure produced by livestock grazing, forests and permanent pastures, and forest litter and organic material that is physically transferred from forest and pastures to the cropped area. In

Management of plant nutrients

IPNS is used to maintain or adjust soil fertility and plant nutrient supply to achieve a given level of crop production. This is done by optimizing the benefits from all possible sources of plant nutrients. The main objectives are to:

- maintain or enhance soil productivity through a balanced use of mineral fertilizers combined with organic and biological sources of plant nutrients;
- improve the stock of plant nutrients in the soil;
- improve the efficiency of plant nutrients, thus limiting losses to the environment.

FAO'S IPNS Approach

IPNS promote the rationalization of the transfer of organic matter and plant nutrients from noncropped areas to cropped areas, and the mobilization of unused nutrient resources or the saving of valuable nutrient sources diverted as domestic fuel, raw materials for building or for industrial purposes. At village level, IPNS also involve the development of the financial capacity of farmers for the adoption of change through farmers' associations.

Plant nutrient balance

An agricultural ecosystem differs from a natural one in that plant nutrients are constantly being removed and exported, and in that sources of plant nutrients outside the cropped area may be used to increase production. In a natural ecosystem, the supply of nutrients at least compensates losses from runoff, leaching and volatilization and, in favourable conditions, nutrients accumulate in the perennial vegetation and in the topsoil. In agricultural systems, farmers intervene at several stages of the plant nutrient cycle in order to optimize crop production and the corresponding export of nutrients.

Farmers try to satisfy plant nutrient demand by using the 'immobilized capital' of plant nutrients in the soil and the 'working capital' of plant nutrients from natural and organic sources. They complement these with external nutrients. However, the nutrients stored in the soil should not be depleted beyond a critical level. These nutrients cannot be transferred rapidly from one plot to another. Plant nutrients in crop residues, manure, litter from forests, green manure and domestic wastes compose a 'working capital' because farmers can transfer them and allocate them to a particular crop in a crop rotation and to a particular plot.

A balance sheet can be established for every nutrient. The efficiency of a production system depends on the importance of crop uptake versus the total supply of nutrients. High losses of nutrients limit the efficiency. Plant nutrient stocks can be 'mined' providing this does not affect the annual supply of nutrients or the general status of soil fertility.

Normally, insufficiency of one plant nutrient limits the efficiency with which other plant nutrients are taken up, reducing crop yield. Unbalanced availability of nutrients can lead to mining of soil reserves for nutrients in short supply and to losses of plant nutrients supplied in excess. Lack of balance also encourages excessive uptake of the nutrients supplied in excess, decreasing the productivity of those nutrients. Unbalanced fertilization is an uneconomic waste of scarce resources.

In practice, the quantity of nutrients available for recycling via plant and animal residues is rarely sufficient to compensate for the amounts removed in agricultural products, even in low-productivity situations. In addition, losses inevitably occur, even in the best-managed systems. Consequently, mineral fertilizers have to play a key role in areas where increased agricultural production is required.

Economic aspects of fertilizer use

Farmers apply plant nutrients only if their effects on crop yields are profitable. The decision to apply external plant nutrients is generally based on economics (price and affordability) but is also conditioned by availability and the production risks involved. The pursuit of higher production has to be balanced against the need to maintain soil fertility and avoid soil degradation.

The profitability of adopting IPNS should, however, be viewed over the long term, since improved efficiency in crop nutrient use tends to become apparent only after several seasons. A number of economic and institutional factors must also be taken into account:

- the price relationship between plant nutrients and the crops to which they are applied, together with the market outlook for these crops, determines how profitable it will be to use fertilizer;
- income and the availability of credit decide whether farmers can afford to buy plant nutrients;
- lack of security of land tenure can reduce the incentive for farmers to use fertilizers.

Small-scale farmers with few resources are compelled to look for short-term results when applying plant nutrients. The removal of access constraints to markets and production technology, and protection from risks, would allow farmers to use plant nutrients economically and in ways that support sustainable crop production.

Advice on efficient plant nutrition

Providing good advice to farmers and enhancing their decision-making capacity is the best way to promote the sustainable intensification of agriculture. Such advice:

- requires a good knowledge of farmers' cropping systems, socio-economic conditions and decisionmaking processes;
- should use farmers' participation to identify and test suitable innovations;
- should be organized in steps from plot level to farm, village territory and small watershed level;
- should include short-term suggestions for the fertilization of crop rotations and longer-term suggestions for accumulating plant nutrients on the farm and improving soil fertility;
- must promote sustainability.

The organization of correct advice is costly and the sharing of this cost among the government, the farmers' communities and the private sector is desirable.

The extent of the study can be defined only after initial discussions with farmers, extension agents and research workers in the area, and a rapid survey of the area. The latter should be conducted by a multidisciplinary team including plant and livestock scientists, social scientists and economists. The study should determine the physical, biological and socio-economic environments, sociocultural characteristics, and production system and land use. Discussions should also be held with farmers to determine their production objectives and constraints, and to get a general idea of their perceptions and living conditions.

Plot level

Advice at plot level should be based on local on-farm experiments. These experiments will provide information on the impact of combined nutrient doses, timing of nutrient supply, and sources of nutrients on crop yields. The experiments should be simple and are of two types: site-specific trials and validation trials. The data collected from the trials are used to derive nutrient response curves for the predominant cropping systems and conditions. These trials are usually managed by public sector researchers because they require a fair degree of control of variability as well as a high level of supervision. Farmer participation in information gathering and decision making is minimal. However, researchers can interact with the farmers and learn about their methods of production. Important considerations in planning site-specific trials are population definition, choice of sites, choice of treatments, experimental designs, and management of the experiment. Sites for the trials should be representative of the farming conditions of the area being studied.

Site-specific, researcher-managed trials

Farmers must be involved in all stages of planning and execution of the trials so that they understand the aims and objectives of the experiment and are willing to participate. Researchers and extension workers must first listen to the farmers' concerns and establish a relationship with the farmer. Farmers must feel that they are equal partners in the experimentation process. The benefits of the research, the importance of farmer participation and the expectations of the relationship must be explained to farmers. Each participant researcher, extension worker and farmer must be apprised of his or her responsibilities who does what, who takes what risks and who gets what products so that all operations are conducted on time and there is no misunderstanding of roles.

All data collected from the trials should be screened, validated, analysed and interpreted by the researchers after completion of the trial. The results obtained will be used to adjust treatments for subsequent trials and to identify promising treatments which can be applied in validation trials.

Validation trials

When promising plant nutrition treatments have been identified, they are tested on farmers' fields in validation trials. Validation trials are conducted by farmers themselves under the overall supervision of extension workers and researchers.

These trials generate valuable information on farmers' understanding, acceptance, rejection, adaptation or adoption of the proposed innovations. The farms should be selected for characteristics (such as slope, integration of livestock and level of management) that are similar to those used for the site-specific trials. The farms should also be representative of all farmers in the area of study both good and bad, so that the range of possible responses to the technology is obtained.

Data generated from these validation trials are screened, validated, analysed and interpreted by extension workers. The data are then compared with the references obtained from the researcher-managed trials to evaluate the farmers' progress and determine possible improvements.

Farm level

Farmers' decisions on how to use plant nutrients depend on the situation of the entire farm and its crop rotation system. Factors taken into consideration include: production objectives, available resources (both fixed and variable, such as land, labour, capital and credit), needs for home consumption, market opportunities and climatic conditions. These factors must be well understood before alternative plant nutrition schemes can be suggested. In addition, advisers must identify the centres of decision making, the organization of land use and crop rotations, and the competing demands for scarce resources such as organic material, labour and capital.

As a first step, an apparent plant nutrient balance inputs versus outputs as well as the practices which may be contributing to nutrient losses or inefficient plant nutrient management should be analysed. This analysis may suggest alternative technologies. The box below gives some potential solutions. Once all potential plant nutrient sources have been identified and possible technologies selected, farmers can determine the correct mix of these technologies to optimize their resource use and meet their production objectives. The new alternatives may involve an increase in labour requirements or financial investments, modification of the farm structure or adaptation of land use and crop rotations. Arrangements will, therefore, need to be made for a complementary supply of external inputs. In particular, attention should be given to farmers' purchasing capacity for these external inputs. The proposed technological package which entails the use of plant nutrients from different sources must be tested to verify its appropriateness to the farmers' situation and to evaluate farmers' acceptance of the technology.

This is done through a network of local pilot farms which is used to evaluate the impact of change on farming conditions. The farms also serve as 'demonstration plots' for neighbouring farmers who may adopt the technology if they see it is to their benefit. In implementing the technology on the pilot farms, farmers must agree on:

- their need to change from their current production system;
- the way in which they and the extension workers will implement the change; and
- mechanisms of risk management during the change.

For these reasons, the choice of farmers and the relationship between farmer and adviser are critical to success. Farmers should be representative of the region and willing to cooperate. Close interaction between extension workers and farmers is needed at all times so that farmers' questions can be answered. This also allows the extension worker to evaluate the farmers response to the technology and find out why they accept or reject it. Sometimes, farmers modify the proposed technology. Extension workers can then determine the reasons for the change and alter treatments in subsequent seasons.

The network of pilot farms should run for at least one entire crop rotation, with the results for each season being used to adjust treatments for subsequent crops. Estimates should be made of crop production and productivity, as well as plant nutrient status, and economic variables such as cash flows, savings and labour inputs. The decision to change the mix of nutrient sources should be guided by whether the benefits of the innovation (both economic and social) outweigh the cost of the investment.

The process of planning, implementing and evaluating change at the farm level is costly and requires a cadre of trained researchers and extension workers, and costly equipment. It can therefore be done only through a limited series of case studies. These can then be used to generate guidelines, methods and reference material which can be adapted by other researchers and extension workers for their specific situations.

Village level

In many traditional low input/low output farming systems, plant nutrition management relies on local nutrient resources collected in areas other than those farmed. Development of an efficient plant nutrition management system should, therefore, extend beyond the farm to the village territory. The main considerations at the village level are:

- management of the transfer of plant nutrients from non-cropped to cropped areas;
- investments for soil and water conservation and their impact on plant nutrient efficiency;
- the effect of poor plant nutrition management practices on the village community; and
- farmers' groups and organizations.

Plant nutrients from non-cropped areas include litter from forests and fodder from pastures. Improving the transfer of these materials to the cropped area can enhance the plant nutrient content in the cropped area.

Some examples of improved management practices include the cultivation of leguminous forest species, alley cropping of forests with pasture crops, mineral fertilization of pastures, regulation of bush fires and development of systems for allocating manure produced by collective herds.

Soil and water conservation can greatly reduce losses of plant nutrients through runoff and leaching. In addition, water harvesting techniques and the development of irrigation will lead to increased efficiency of nutrient use. These investments require the cooperation of the entire village and must therefore be considered while developing efficient plant nutrition management systems.

Poor plant nutrient management by individual farmers results in a decrease in soil fertility because of heavy mining, erosion, silting and deforestation. Similarly, an oversupply of nutrients may pollute drinking water and poor management of organic wastes is a potential heath hazard. Thus the involvement of sound plant nutrient management by the entire farming community is essential in developing a system at the village level.

At the village level, farmers' groups can create favourable conditions for the procurement of inputs and access to credit. Farmers' associations, trade connections between these associations and the input sector as well as traders in agricultural products and banks should therefore be encouraged to support improved plant nutrition management by farmers.

Advice on quantities of nutrients to be applied may be based on empirical results from field experiments, on soil or plant analysis, on a nutrient balance-sheet approach, on mathematical models of nutrient dynamics, or on a combination of methods. In the absence of more detailed information, knowledge of the quantities of nutrients removed by crops at the desired yield level provides a starting point for estimating nutrient requirements.

Field experiments are valuable in providing quantitative information on the supply of nutrients from soil and organic residues, and the short-term effects on crop yield from mineral fertilizers supplied in different forms and quantities. This provides a vital basis for advising farmers and for testing and improving advice systems.

Wherever possible, long-term field experiments should be set up so that residual effects of fertilizers and organic sources on crop growth and soil properties can be studied and taken into account when formulating nutrient recommendations. Such experiments can also provide information on interactions between nutrient applications and other agricultural activities, and on the likelihood of unforeseen problems such as environmental contamination or deficiency of a secondary or micronutrient. In this context, the need for balanced plant nutrition should be emphasized.

Research organizations are responsible for informing the public about the innovations and their potential impact.

Many people are concerned about the possible side effects of plant nutrients on the environment. This concern refers both to the use of mineral fertilizers and organic sources of nutrients, the latter in connection with intensive livestock farming that leads to the production of so much organic waste that it cannot be used effectively, converted or disposed of. Four important issues have to be highlighted:

- Fertilizers are often referred to as agrochemicals, a term which groups plant nutrients with insecticides, herbicides and fungicides. A clear distinction must be made between fertilizers, which provide nutrients that are essential for plant growth, and biocides, compounds that kill, which are used for plant protection.
- The environmental effects of applying plant nutrients can be positive or negative, and statements on the issue should be objectively balanced.
- The amounts of plant nutrients, both mineral and organic, that are applied in developing countries are relatively low. Local excesses in some industrial countries should not prejudice increased agricultural production in the developing world.
- Environmental problems related to the application of

plant nutrients depend less on the nature of the nutrients than on the amounts and the way they are applied. Detrimental effects are mostly due to overdoses or to improper or unbalanced use that can be corrected by improved management practices. The positive effects are summarized in the box below and the negative effects in the text that follows.

Negative effects with high inputs

Not all nutrients applied to the soil are taken up by the growing crop and the remainder may become an environmental hazard. Unused nutrients can remain in the soil, be removed in water leaching through the soil or in runoff, or be lost to the atmosphere by volatilization. The relative importance of these phenomena depends on the physico-chemical and biological reactions in which the nutrients take part.

Environmental issues

- efficient use of plant nutrients ensures that yields are higher than those obtained on the basis of inherent soil fertility by correcting either an overall deficiency or an imbalance of nutrients;
- nutrients removed from the soil through harvesting and export of produce can be replenished in order to maintain and enhance production potential;
- by increasing yields per unit area on good arable land, plant nutrients allow land of low quality, for example land susceptible to erosion, to be withdrawn from cultivation and reduce overall pressure on the land, including deforestation and overgrazing of non-cropped areas;
- plant nutrients ease the problem of erosion control on cropped areas because of the protection provided by a dense and vigorous crop cover;
- IPNS promote the correct management of plant

nutrients on the farm and the watershed, optimizing the economic value of the nutrients and limiting nutrient losses to the environment.

Positive Environmental Effects of Plant Nutrients

Nitrogen: under normal farming conditions, on welldrained soils and with favourable temperature conditions, all soluble nitrogen compounds are fairly rapidly oxidized to nitrate. Nitrate is not absorbed to any appreciable extent by soil particles. Nitrogen is therefore the most likely fertilizer element to be leached out into surface water or groundwater, or to be lost to the atmosphere by denitrification, partly as nitrogen gas and partly as nitrous oxide, which is a greenhouse gas. Nitrate derived from the breakdown of organic matter in soil, slurry or manure applied to land is also subject to leaching. In many temperate regions, this is often a more significant source of nitrate than mineral fertilizer. Improved farming practices can help reduce the leaching by maximizing utilization of the nitrate provided by the soil, and applying just the right amount of nitrogen at the right time for each crop. Researchers trying to understand changes in nitrate concentrations in drainage waters should take due account of changes in land use and agricultural practice, as well as fertilizer use.

In industrialized farming systems, intensive animal husbandry is a major cause of the leaching of nitrogen. This is partly due to untimely mineralization of nitrogen from urine, faeces, and manure or slurry. Nitrate produced when crop growth is not vigorous can be the origin of leaching or denitrification. The other main problem is ammonia volatilization, both from manure heaps and from soil soon after manure application. Ammonia can also be volatilized if urea fertilizer is applied to soil of high pH under warm and dry conditions.

Phosphorus: plants are supplied with phosphorus in the form of phosphate ions. They are immobilized in the soil, being strongly adsorbed by the surfaces of iron, aluminium and manganese oxides and hydroxides, and by clay particles. Applied phosphate that is not taken up by the crop remains in the soil unless it is washed off the land by runoff or by soil erosion. Phosphate can also occur in high concentrations in irrigation water and drainage water from inundated soils. Excess inputs of phosphates to surface waters can lead to eutrophication and algal blooms.

Plant nutrients are supplied from sources such as mineral fertilizer, the soil, rainfall and dust, irrigation water and biofixation. As the graph shows. the contributions of these sources are cumulative.

The crop takes up a portion of the available nitrogen, regardless of its origin. Available nitrogen not taken up by the plant is lost to the environment. This loss is the difference between the total available and the total uptake the difference between the top line of the biofixation block and the relevant uptake curve.

At low levels of supplied N, there is little uptake and so the loss of N to the environment is high. As the nitrogen supply increases, the plant takes up more of the nitrogen until it cannot increase its uptake any further. Supplying additional nitrogen results in increased losses to the environment. Plant nutrient loss is minimized at the point where the distance between the uppermost line and the uptake curve is smallest. For a crop with a low level of uptake, the minimum loss of nitrogen is the difference (a-c). For a higher level of uptake, the minimum loss is (a-b). These minima occur at the ecological optimum level of N supply. To increase nutrient efficiency (uptake), farmers should practise IPNS and optimize all other production factors.

Phosphate fertilizers may contain cadmium when sedimentary rock phosphate is used as raw material. Cadmium is also added to the soil by aerial deposition. Current fertilizer usage presents no immediate hazard. However, cadmium should be removed when raw materials are processed, wherever possible.

Potassium: potassium ions, in addition to being taken up by plants, are adsorbed by the soil and can even be fixed within clay particles. Added potassium that is not taken up by the crop is therefore not very mobile in soils that contain clay. In sandy soils, some applied potassium may be leached out. Major losses of potassium are caused when the element is washed away in liquid manure from farmyards and dairies. Potassium in water has no detrimental effects but may indicate the presence of sewage or animal effluent. Potassium is not a major factor in the eutrophication of surface waters.

Negative effects with low inputs

Soil fertility: the constant removal of produce without or with insufficient replenishment of plant nutrients causes a steady decline of soil fertility. This mining of plant nutrients, leading to severe depletion of soil fertility, is a major environmental hazard in a number of developing countries.

Land expansion: if land and labour are available, low yields resulting from nutrient depletion force farmers to expand cultivated land, often at the expense of forested areas or marginal soils subject to erosion or desertification.

Amendments: large areas in the tropics are inherently poor in soil nutrients and suffer from acidity and aluminium toxicity. Organic recycling does not offer a solution since the biomass produced in such soils is itself extremely poor in essential plant nutrients. These soils cannot be made productive without amendments and a basic input of plant nutrients. Low or zero use of plant nutrients on such soils prevents the development of agricultural production on a sustained basis.

Overcoming the negative effects

The negative effects of applications of plant nutrients, both at low and high levels of input, can be avoided or remedied by good management. Balanced fertilization should overcome the hazards of nutrient depletion and of mining soil fertility. Judicious management of plant nutrients can prevent pollution, mainly through practices that reduce losses of nutrients to aquifers or the atmosphere. These practices include balanced, timely, targeted fertilization combined with other practices (such as improved varieties, water management and plant protection) that stimulate maximum uptake of plant nutrients by the crop. Due attention should also be given to controlling losses from soil erosion and runoff, and through appropriate land management.

Long-term planning and monitoring of the use of plant nutrients must reconcile four objectives:

- agronomic and economic efficiency to maximize agricultural output from available nutrients;
- increasing the production capacity of the natural resource base;
- consistency with a country's overall economic and environmental goals;
- safeguarding social security and equity for rural populations.

Assessment: efficient assessment of plant nutrient requirements is the basis for planning and for deciding on levels of domestic production and imports of fertilizer products and raw materials, including the use of foreign exchange to finance imports. Fertilizer demand projection is simply an assessment of the plant nutrient volumes that will be ordered by farmers and which are needed to correct any imbalances.

Marketing: marketing systems should promote efficient fertilizer use and satisfy farmers' requirements while helping meet national food self-reliance goals. These systems require careful design and policies that strike the right balance between government and private participation in the production, import and distribution of fertilizers. This is a critical issue that is highly dependent on national economic and political conditions.

Transport and storage: transport and storage are part of the essential infrastructure needed for the efficient use of fertilizers. Costs will partly determine the need for alternative means of transport, and the location and size of storage facilities.

Training: demonstrations, training and extension on efficient crop-production and fertilizer-use techniques are essential components of farm-support policies. Extension requirements must be assessed and services established to address the technological level and experience of the farming community. Adequate technological packages, including the balanced use of mineral fertilizers as part of an IPNS, and basic knowledge of the economics of fertilizer use have to be introduced.

Pricing: price is an important factor in improving the income of farmers. Whether or not to subsidize the product or the inputs in order to stimulate production has long been a controversial issue. Most developing countries in Asia have used input subsidies in agriculture; developed countries support farm activities with other mechanisms, often with indirect or invisible effects, and not always to stimulate production. Subsidies given directly or indirectly to farmers for fertilizers have been the most important pricing factor in developing countries. They have been clearly shown to

Policies for effective plant nutrition

Policies for effective plant nutrition should address the following topics:

- determining the balance between domestic food production and food imports for countries aiming at food self-reliance;
- assessing plant nutrient requirements;
- choosing the sources and combinations of plant nutrient supplies;
- determining domestic production and imports of fertilizer products and raw materials;

- setting price levels for nutrients vis-à-vis the price of produce;
- providing distribution, marketing and credit facilities, including adequate foreign exchange allocation;
- legislation; and
- supporting extension and research (access to technology).

Legislation: fertilizer legislation deals mostly with specifications on composition, in terms of nutrients and inert material, concentration of plant nutrients, physical properties, package characteristics, labelling and weight, storage and quality control.

Packaging: fertilizer packaging should reduce losses but not add substantially to the price of fertilizer. It should also convey the right information to users. Fertilizer distribution systems and requirements for storage and transport condition the quality of fertilizer packaging. The chemical and physical properties of the products and conditions of storage, especially at the end of the distribution chain, must also be considered.

Advice and planning should involve both government and the private sector. A focal point for fertilizer advice and planning is needed to establish a well-integrated fertilizer policy, coordinated with the country's agricultural and food-security policies, and in harmony with national priorities. This focal point can also advise on prices and marketing policy, and be responsible for demand forecasting and identifying research and extension priorities.

Financing: fertilizer is a product for which demand is often highly seasonal. Fertilizer traders' cash flow is therefore highly variable and traders will need commercial credit in foreign and domestic currency.

4

BIOCHAR-- Its Role in Crop Nutrition

Agriculture is of climate change relevance due to emissions in food production, and emissions through land-use change. Globally, these account for carbon-equivalent emissions equal to that of transport. Since agricultural emissions are affected by fertiliser application and the extent of the livestock sector, emissions are - as for transport - expected to increase at a faster rate then population growth *per se*, as a function of wealth creation and dietary change. However, the fact that agricultural land is actively managed means that the emissions can potentially be mitigated, or reversed. Agricultural soils contain a relatively small proportion of the global soil pool, but the C contained in those is large relative to the annual atmospheric C flux. Biochar comprises biomass that is a deliberately stabilised form of C, for which the soil may provide storage on a very large scale. Due to certain physical and chemical properties of some biochars, these forms of carbon can offer potential value to crop productivity through interactions with nutrients and soil mineral particles. Any improvement to the productivity of existing agricultural land has the potential to ease pressure on bio-diverse and often carbon-rich natural ecosystems. It is in this context that biochar has emerged as a potential win–win strategy for climate change mitigation and food production at the global scale. Producing charcoal using traditional kilns liberates greenhouse gases, particularly methane and nitrous oxide, and conserves relatively small propositions of carbon in the feedstock and wastes the heat energy product. As well as being associated with deforestation, sequestration of carbon into charcoal using unmodified, traditional methods may not (depending on the source and ordinary fate of feedstock) provide climate change mitigation. Controlled pyrolysis, on the other hand, stabilises biomass carbon in solid form but also captures energy-rich liquids and gases which can be used to drive the pyrolysis reactions or used for energy elsewhere. Applying biochar to agricultural soil is proposed for three reasons: (1) only the soil seems to have a capacity sufficient to accommodate biochar at the scale relevant to the long-term mitigation of climate change, (2) there is potential for biochar to enhance soil function, and (3) a suppression of methane and nitrous oxide release increases the value of biochar as a means to offset agricultural greenhouse gas emissions.

Ideally biochar will provide reliable agronomic benefits and command a value in crop production that precludes combustion for energy, with or without a value placed on sequestration of the carbon that it contains. In this evaluation of value, allowance has to be made for the cost of acquisition and incorporation of biochar into soil. A value can also be assigned by producers and upstream food processors to the marketing potential of low-carbon or "carbon neutral" food products produced in systems that deploy biochar. It is expected that growing understanding of the relationship between feedstock, the manipulation of the pyrolysis process and the function of biochar in soil will ultimately enable biochar to be "engineered" to provide the balance of benefits most appropriate to a particular system. The value of the energy captured in pyrolysis must also exceed the price for the alternative use of the feedstock, unless it is genuinely a waste, in which case the normal cost of disposal can be added to the value of the energy. It should be recognised that the price of feedstock depends on demand. Wastes may cease to be wastes once demand for their use as feedstock exceeds their rate of production within the relevant catchment. In a closed cycle biochar system, biochar is incorporated into the same land, the same enterprise, or groups of enterprises from which the pyrolysis feedstock originates. A typical scenario would involve the use of cereal crop straw that, in intensive arable areas, is often available at relatively low cost. The typical yield of straw in high yielding systems is up to 2 t C ha-1. A key advantage of a biochar strategy is that, assuming that the provision of key functions is limited only by the longevity of the biochar, its stability would dictate that the application frequency required to deliver benefits are single or occasional, rather than annual. The proximity of a pyrolysis facility to an adequate catchment for feedstock must be economically and logistically viable, and can potentially affect the CO_2 - equivalent savings. This is the case for biomass and bioenergy facilities generally. However, for biochar the proximity of suitable locations for biochar application to soil is important as well. If the gathering of feedstock and distribution of biochar occur over the same area the logistical and cost impacts may not be greatly affected.

Possible off-farm sources of pyrolysis feedstock include municipal green waste (from gardens and parks), composted urban waste, digested sewage sludge, mixed municipal waste. In addition, in the future by-products of other bioenergy or bio-fuel systems are likely to become available. Utilising off-farm wastes is attractive in cost terms where it results in avoided landfill and other disposal costs. In addition, compared to typical or existing disposal methods, there may be a lower emission of CH_4 and N_2O greenhouse gases than placement in soil, enhancing the net gain in carbon equivalents through avoided emissions of gases with much higher global warming potential. However, many such wastes have a high water content which will incur increased emissions (and cost) associated with higher requirement for process energy in pyrolysis.

Studies conducted during the 1980s and 1990s tended to

show marked impacts of low charcoal additions on various crop species, but inhibition at higher rates. Since then, data has been published for a number of other field experiments where the short-term response of staple grain crops to biochar application, in terms of plant biomass or crop yield, has been assessed. Positive yield effects from biochar addition were reported by Kimetu who was able to establish that the impact was in part due to non-nutrient improvement to soil function. Improved fertiliser use efficiency was pinpointed as an explanation for biochar maintaining yields after forest clearance in Amazonia, in essentially a recreation of *terra preta*. Biochar-amended plots receiving NPK sustained higher crop yield compared to control plots where yield declined rapidly. Results from semi-arid soils in Australia have shown positive response to biochar in combination with fertiliser in pot trials and in Indonesia maize and peanut yields were enhanced where bark charcoal was applied in combination with N fertiliser in the field. The view that nutrient management and pre-existing soil nutrient status determine crop response to biochar was supported by a study in rice, where statistically higher first-season yield was observed only when biochar (at a low rate) was appiied together with fertiliser N and in a low-yielding crop variety; yield was lower than the control in an equivalent treatment using a high yielding and thus N-demanding variety. Low rates of application in an Australian study in wheat suggested that significant fertiliser savings can be obtained through biochar additions. A pot study of maize showed higher biological nitrogen fixation with biochar addition due to nutrient effects higher yield and N uptake reported in pot trials using radish. A key consideration highlighted in several studies is the potential for biochar to immobilise previously plant available N. This could be from the mineralisation of labile, high C-to-N fractions of biochar drawing N into microbial biomass, sorption of ammonium, or sequestration of soil solution into fine pores.

The mechanisms of crop response are difficult to assess in the absence of long-term data. Development of predictive certainty for the longevity and durability of yield and other effects, particularly in relation to specific crop and soil types, is critical to guide selection of feedstock, production method, and application rate. Predictability and certainty are required to assign a financial value to the agronomic value of biochar, and to open the possibility for large scale deployment.

5

Silicon Nutrition and Crop Production

Introduction

Per acre yield of most of agricultural crops in Pakistan is very low compared to many of the other countries. Among the factors responsible for low yield, biotic stresses insect pest and disease attack and a-biotic stresses are very important. Crop species differ greatly for their tolerance and or resistance against these stresses because of different genetic characteristics. Environmental factors may be mineral nutrition contribute considerably in increasing and or decreasing the plant's resistance and or tolerance against these stresses.

Integrated nutrient management practices are gaining popularity nowadays and management of 13 physiologically essential nutrients namely six macro nutrients and seven micronutrients is generally considered by the agronomists for sustaining and increasing crop yields. However, there are some elements that under certain agro-clirnatic conditions enhance plant growth by promoting several physiological processes but are not essential. Although not considered essential, these elements are said to be beneficial nutrient.

Silicon is an example of such elements.

The maintenance of photosynthetic activity due to Si fertilization could be one of the reasons for increased dry matter production in rice crop. Disease severity or incidence tends to be reduced with increasing tissue contents of Si in rice in cotton and in sugarcane. This review intends to summarize the potential agroeconomic benefits of Si inclusion in integrated nutrient management.

Silicon Nutrition of Crops

Silicon is the second most abundant element in the earth's crust, with soils containing approximately 32 percent Si by weight. The essentiality of Si as a nutrient for higher plants is very difficult to prove because of its ubiquitous presence in the biosphere. Even highly purified water contains about 20 nM Si. Different species and varieties within species utilize greatly different amounts of Si from the growth medium. The plant absorbs Si from the solution in the form of mono silicic acid which has no electric charge and is not very much mobile in plant. Movement of Si follows that of water as the uptake of H4Si04 is nonselective and energetically passive and its transport from root to shoot is in the transpiration stream in the xylem. In rice, however, large amount of Si in leaves cannot be fully explained by the passive uptake and may be active by gaining energy from the anaerobic respiration (van del' Vorrn, 1980), Silicon deposited in the walls of epidermal cells after absorption by plants, contributes considerably to stem strength.

Monosilicic acid polymerizes to Si gel when Si concentration increases in the plant water or biogenetic opal as amorphous Si02.nH20. Transpiration rate of the specific part determines the distribution of Si within the shoot and shoot parts of plant. The epidermal cell walls become effective barriers against both fungal infections and water loss by cuticular transpiration when impregnated with a firm Si layer.

Silicon is not much mobile element in plants therefore, a

continued supply of this element would be required particularly for healthy and productive development of plant during all growth stages. In a field study, plant height was quadratically related to the rate of Si application, while it related linearly with crop plant stem diameter. In another solution culture experiment shoot dry matter of cotton plants increased three fold with Si application as compared to control, In a nutrient culture experiment, the application of Si decreased the uptake of N, K, Fe and Mn in transplanted rice and increased the uptake of P, Ca, Mg and the formation of carbohydrate.

In short, Si is a beneficial element for most of the crop plants especially for rice and sugarcane. The potential beneficial effects of Si for most of the crops are summarized here.

Potential Benefits of Silicon Nutrition

The effective management of Si can offer several potential benefits for crop production including improved plant growth, increased yield, induced resistance to stresses and increased productivity of problem soils.

Improved Plant Growth and Yield

Low per acre yield of most of crops is common in developing countries like Pakistan and imbalanced nutrition is one of the most important causes for this low yield. Research work demonstrating the effects of Si on yield of various crops especially rice and sugarcane is well documented in few areas of world especially USA, Brazil and Japan. The yield responses are great enough that Si fertilization in rice and sugarcane is a common practice in these countries.

Silicon nutrition has several beneficial effects on plant growth largely due to its unique physiological role. Adatia and Besford reported a number of positive effects of Si on the growth of cucumber plants such as more leaf thickness, more dry matter per unit area of leaf, a small but significant added increment in root fresh and dry weight, and less propensity of leaves to wilt. In another experiment, Si application to growth medium significantly improved growth of cotton plants infected with root rot. The shoot dry matter increased about three fold and root dry matter about two fold due to Si application. Formation of new roots was also observed in cotton plants as Si was added to the nutrient solution, when earlier roots were rotted due to uncertain causes. In dense stand of cereals, low light intensity is likely to limit photosynthesis; the modifying effect of Si on leaf erectness can be beneficial. The maintenance of photosynthetic activity due to Si fertilization could be one of the reasons for the increased dry matter production. They also observed an increase in water use efficiency in Si amended rice plants probably due to prevention of excessive transpiration.

In various field experiments, various slags applied to nursery plants increased the number of leaves and dry matter of rice plants. After transplanting, Si fertilization increased the number of tillers and panicles. The function of Si deposition in cell walls is analogous of that of lignin. Silicon prevents the compression of xylem vessel when transpiration is high. In experiments with both in solutions culture and soil grown plants, a recurring observation has been that plants supplied with sufficient Si resist lodging. The mechanical strength of plants resides in cell wall, which enables them to maintain an erect habit.

Reviews on the role of Si in plants, therefore. stress the association of Si with cell walls and discuss the increased rigidity of cell walls of plants grown with ample available Si in terms of that association. Savant et al. reported several levels of yield increases due to Si application in rice and sugarcane. When Si is applied, yield increases of 10 % are common in rice and exceed 30 % when leaf blast is severe. The benefits of Si ferti lization are generally observed in rice and sugarcane grown on weathered tropical soils and Histosols, which are Si deficient. Gascho and Andreis concluded that Si is a beneficial and probably essential for sugarcane grown on organic and quartz sand soils. Increases in tonnage of sugarcane amounting to 18 % in cane and 22 % in sugar for plant cane crop after the application of electric furnace slag to Latosols has been reported by Ayers (1966). This beneficial effect of slag on low Si soils lasted for four years.

Induced Resistance to Stresses

Biotic stresses such as pests and plant diseases, and abiotic stresses such as soil water shortage, salinity and mineral toxicities, etc, are very common under field conditions reducing crop yields drastically. Silicon has a unique physiological role in alleviating both biotic and abiotic stresses in most of the crops.

Biotic Stresses

Silicon can reduce the severity of several important diseases of rice, including blast, brown spot, sheath blight, leaf scald and grain discoloration and of sugarcane, including leaf freckling and ring spot. Fungal hyphae and parasite hustoria successfully infecting plant cells must break the cell wall, which they do through chemical means. Formation of a physical barrier in epidermal cells by Si deposition contributes to plant resistance against diseases and pests. Rodrigues et al. reported a significant reduction in sheath blight development in rice with the addition of Si. 1n another experiment, Rodrigues et al., reported that Si fertilization increased the host resistant against sheath blight III nee.

In most disease control programmes fungicides and or resistant cultivars are being used. However, host resistance may not always be practical and when available can breakdown due to shifts in pathogen races. Fungicides are currently perceived to be potentially harmful to the environment, particularly to the soil and water. Therefore, an encouraging alternative to fungicide use is Si fertilization offering an enhancement in resistance of host plant against these stresses. Deren et al. concluded that the increase in rice yield with added Si was attributable to increased resistance against diseases such as brown spot, being negatively correlated with Si concentration in the plant tissue. In Brazil, Korndorfer et al. found that an increase in Si application rate reduced grain discoloration from 46% in the control to 29% at the highest Si rate, it was also found that this difference corresponds to a 64% reduction in grain discoloration. In other field experiment at Florida, Seebold et al. reported that the number of sporolating lesions, lesion size, rate of lesion expansion, diseased leaf area, and number of spores per lesions reduced with increasing rate of Si applicaiton. Silicon deposited in the epidermal tissue mechanically deters hyphae invasion. Furthermore, Si physiologically promotes ammonium assimilation and restrains the increase in soluble N compounds, including amino acids and amide, which are instrumental for the propagation of hyphae.

The presence of Si crystals in epidermal tissues hinder the feeding of the insect, which in their phase has rather fragile mandibles. Plants like sugarcane and rice, with high Si content, seem to interfere in the feeding of larvae, damaging their mandibles. It is possible that plants with higher Si contents in their tissue would have a higher level of resistance to the infections by such pests.

Abiotic Stresses

The climate of Pakistan is arid and semi arid and water stress in fields is common effecting crop yields significantly. Silicon significantly improves water economy of plants largely by reducing cuticular transpiration. Excessive rate of transpiration is one of the symptoms associated with Si deficiency. In nutrient culture experiment, the wilted cotton plants became erect when Si was added. This erectness may be attributed to improved water economy and hinders the root xylem to rupture due to excessive transpiration. The rate of transpiration is presumably influenced by the amount of Si gel associated with the cellulose in the cell walls of epidermal cells. Hence, a well-thickened layer of Si gel should help to retard water loss, while epidermal cell wall with less Si gel will allow water to escape at an accelerated rate.

Salinity restricts the growth of crops hence holds back the development of sustainable agriculture. By increasing Si content of plants, it may be possible to reduce plant's internal water stress and thereby enable them to withstand salt stress. A less decrease in shoot dry matter accumulation of salt stressed barley plants when Si was added to growth medium can be attributed to increased CO2 assimilation and decreased electrolyte leakage and Na concentration in shoot.

Promotion in dry biomass of wheat under saline conditions can also be described as a function of increased water influx. which apart from preventing physiological drought may help to maintain a balanced and efficient absorption and translocation of mineral elements required for energy generations. There may be a possibility of an interaction between freely available Na and Si ions, forming a complex, which reduce their transportation to the aerial parts of plants. They observed low amounts of Si on the flag leaves at 0.6% NaCI with Si treatment, which may be attributed to the binding of soluble Si with Na in root and retarding its upward translocation. In solution culture experiment, Liang et al., found that Si could enhance the uptake of K and inhibit the uptake of Na by salt stressed barley, thus mitigating the toxicity of salt to barley and increasing salt tolerance of the plants.

Lodging can be defined as bending and or breaking over of a plant before its harvest resulting in economic loss to farmers by lowering the quantity and quality of yield. Increased plant Si content has been reported to increase mechanical strength of plant tissue, which resultd in reduced lodging. Lee et al. also noticed an increase in resistance to lodging due to application of Si fertilizer to rice. Liang et al. reported less than 10 % or practically no lodging in rice fields fertilized with a new silicate material and more than 60 % lodging in control fields. Evidently, thickening of cell walls of the sclerenchyma tissue in the clum and or shortening and thickening of internodes or increase in Si content of lower internodes provides mechanical strength to enable plant to resist lodging. Under field conditions, particularly in dense stands of cereals, Si can stimulate growth and yield by decreasing mutual shading through improved leaf erectness. Leaf erectness is an important factor affecting light interception in dense plant population and, hence, photosynthesis. This effect of Si on leaf erectness is mainly a function of the Si deposition in the epidermal layer of the leaf panicle. Thakahashi has reviewed that Si increased the oxidizing power of rice roots. The roots of rice supplied with Si shows a higher oxidation power of ferrous' iron than of non-supplied one. Due to a decrease in the solubility of iron caused by iron oxidation, the Si supplied rice absorbs less Iron.

Silicon is also reported to alleviate Mn toxicity. Adding Si to the solution did not diminish to Mn content of the leaves. Rather. in the absence of Si, Mn was concentrated in necrotic spots, whereas in the presence of Si, the Mn was distributed more evenly in leaves and thus preventing it from collecting into localized areas which became necrotic. Aluminum toxicity is also reported to be alleviated by Si application.

6

Balanced Crop Nutrition: Fertilizing for Crop and Food Quality

Outcome of unbalanced crop nutrition

This paper presents 4 different country examples of negative K balances. In India, the slow but continuous reduction in the soil's K supply in the Indo-Gangetic plains may lead to stagnating or reduced yields. In China, the demand for K in regions with highly weathered soils and an insufficient K supply, when accompanied by a positive balance for N and P, causes a large negative K balance. In Egypt, on the highly productive irrigated land there is a severe negative K balance, especially on soils of low fertility. In Bulgaria, a recent assessment of farm gate and regional nutrient balances shows a decline in soil fertility.

Yadvinder-Singh et al. studied the long-term effects of organic inputs on yield and soil fertility in the typical rice-wheat crop rotation practiced in the Indo- Gangetic plains in India. After the dramatic rise in productivity during the 1970s and early 1980s, yields in this region have either remained stagnant or declined. Yields of cereals in the Punjab are the largest in India and they receive the most nutrients (368 kg ha-1), yet with very little K of only about 10 kg ha-1.

The detailed balance calculation of input output for K showed that over a 12-year period the negative K balance varied between -932 and -1810 kg K ha-1, depending on the treatment and consequent yield and K input through straw and farmyard manure.

The addition of K through organic matter appears to be significant, yet it is not sufficient to supply and replenish the K removed. The balance calculation shows that for a zero net balance an additional ~90 kg K ha-1 year-1 as fertilizer would have been sufficient for both crops (wheat and rice).

Such a negative balance may lead to a decrease in exchangeable potassium in soil. Figure 4 shows the long-term effects of applying no K in the Control + 150N treatment. There has been a decrease of approximately 30% in Kex, as compared to the application of FYM + 150N, which showed only a slight reduction. The authors comment that "Current K fertilizer recommendations for P and K are inadequate in the long run" and they also rule out the possibility of decline in soil organic matter as the reason for negative yield trends. Finally the authors conclude that the adverse changes in climate along with a decreased soil supply of available K may be the possible reasons associated with yield decline.

China

The spatial and temporal variability of N, P, and K balances for agro-ecosystems in China was described by Shen et al. (2005). Inputs of nutrients in fertilizers and organic matter (from crop residues and human and animal excreta) were calculated and compared with their removal in harvested produce. Balances were calculated at province level, which represent the major agroecosystems of China.

Low fertilizer input alone appeared to be the main reason for the K deficit in Xinjiang and Beijing. However, in the Eastern Provinces the negative K balance was due to too small a K input even though it was quite large to replenish the large amount of K removed in the harvested crops and losses by leaching. In addition, large areas of East and Southeast China suffer from a negative K balance ranging from 48 to 72 kg K ha-1 year-1. Interestingly, these provinces are also associated with large surplus applications of N, which aggravate the negative K balance.

The authors related the nutrient balances to economic and social factors. They pointed to the correlation between GOVA per capita gross output of value of agriculture, especially in North China and to NIRH per capita net income of rural households. The lower these socio-economic factors are, the higher is the negative K balance. These findings demonstrate the important role of socio-economic development on nutrient balances.

Egypt

Potassium fertilization in Egyptian irrigated agriculture has become very important since the completion of the High Dam in Aswan, which prevented the continuous deposition on farmers' fields of the Nile silt-rich in K bearing minerals. In addition, Nile alluvial soils with high clay content can have a high K fixing capacity. Thus, even with a high Kex level there might not be sufficient available K for various crops. In addition, the newly reclaimed soils are sandy and calcareous, and poor in organic matter and macro- and micronutrients.

Using the average yields in 2002-2004 of rice, wheat, fruit, and vegetables, the amount of K removed was calculated. Approximately 250,000 mt K2O conservative calculation, with all straw of rice and wheat returned to the field and 489,650 mt K2O with all straw of rice and wheat removed from the field are removed annually.

The production of fruit and vegetables is considerable and therefore very significant in K2O consumption. We estimate that currently these crops are responsible for approximately half of the K2O removed in Egypt. In future, with increased production of fruit and vegetables on the newly reclaimed land, with its poor Ksupplying capacity, there should be a need for higher K2O consumption.

Bulgaria

Nutrient consumption in Bulgaria was at its peak during the mid 1980s, but fell dramatically to about 20%, 0%, and 0% for N, P2O5, and K2O of its peak use during the mid and late 1990s. During this period, fruit production fell by 75%, vegetables by 30%, and cereals by 20%.

Nikolova calculated K balances at farm gate, regional, and national levels. Only dairy farms showed a positive K balance. Arable and mixed farms in 7 regions of Bulgaria, representing all types of soils and regions, all showed a negative K balance due to the very small amounts of K applied. The author concludes that the mean annual K deficiency varies between 43 and 79 kg ha-1, and the national K balance is approximately -200,000 mt K year-1, a similar level since the 1990s.

The long-term consequences of a negative K balance on soil fertility are obvious. In 13 years (1989-2002), the frequency of "Low" K status soils doubled and that of "High" K status fell from 71% to 27%. The following examples demonstrate various consequences of correcting unbalanced nutrient management. These are related to i) long-term fertilization; ii) organic agriculture; iii) the effect of balanced fertilization on yields, quality, and pest and disease infestation and iv) the economics of balanced fertilization.

Long-term observations

Fertilization is a decision taken by the farmer according to economic parameters. When there is no short-term economic response to applied K, the farmer tends to eliminate this factor from his manuring policy. In a 3-year experiment in cotton grown on vermicultic soil, an increase in cumulative yield in the order of 13% to 21% was found for applying 120-240 kg K ha-1; however, at 480 kg K ha-1, an increase of 42% was achieved. These data may mislead, because in 1985 there was only a very small increase in yield from the applied K compared to that of 1987. In addition, application of 480 kg K ha-1 was the only rate in which yields were increasing in all 3 years. In contrast to the large K application, where no K was applied there was a decrease in organic matter and of available soil K that caused K fixation and resulting in a 3- year downward trend in yields. This example illustrates the need to consider the longer-term effect of repeated K fertilization, especially with high K rates in heavy soils with fixation capacity.

Organic agriculture

Organic agriculture is often perceived as a clear-cut solution for better crop production. A mixture of beliefs and scientific data hinders the real questions and consequences from long-term practice of organic agriculture. Can organic farming match today's large requirements for balanced and timely nutrient application? Soil fertility status after 21 years of organic agriculture shows a greater decline in available K in soil than where fertilizers have been used.

A 21-year long-term experiment at Forschungsinstitut für biologischen Landbau in Frick, Switzerland, compares 4 farming systems differing mainly in the management of fertilization and plant protection. Four basic treatments were compared organic systems biodynamic and bioorganic that used farmyard manure and slurry corresponding to a certain amount of livestock per area unit; 1 conventional system using the same amount of farmyard manure as the organic systems but with the addition of mineral fertilizers to reach the plant-specific Swiss standard recommendation; and another conventional system using no fertilizer during the first crop rotation, then mineral fertilizers exclusively, as in regular non-livestock farming.

The results show that yields of winter wheat, potatoes, and grass clover were 20% higher with the 2 non-organic treatments by an amount corresponding to lower input costs, including fuel. However, there was a negative K balance with the organic treatment, compared to a positive balance with mineral NPK. There was a negative N balance with all 4 systems but it was larger with the organic systems compared to that with mineral NPK fertilizers.

In contrast, organic dairy farms have reported positive nutrient balances, mainly due to larger inputs of nutrients in animal feed. Timely application of nutrients from organic sources is complicated. Nitrogen supply is highly dependent on mineralization of the organic matter, which can be assessed in terms of total N supply, but for practical reasons is usually insufficient to meet the requirements of a crop at the appropriate time. Dahlin et al. discussed the use of N from organic material. They showed that the expected leaching loss of N from poultry manure is far greater than that from ammonium nitrate and that N uptake from ammonium nitrate is much higher than that from red clover manure. Clearly, the precise timing and split application of ammonium nitrate can supply N in a much more controllable way than can be achieved with organic materials.

However, efficiency of phosphate use from single superphosphate or poultry litter compost was equal. Even greater efficiency of phosphate use is achieved with fertigation systems, when P is added in very frequent applications of water and fertilizer. In fact, both P and K efficiency were increased by daily and even more frequent application of water and nutrients.

In summary, organic agriculture may cause soil nutrient mining due to insufficient nutrient application and may lead to large losses, especially of nitrogen and potassium, but not necessarily in dairy farms. In contrast, using mineral fertilizers that can be applied at flexible timing and rates can increase the uptake of nutrients and thus reduce loss to the environment.

Effect on yields, quality, and plant health Nutrient application is highly unbalanced in Punjab. In 2004/05, the state consumed 1.562 Mt of nutrients, of which 1.2; 0.32 and 0.043 Mt was N, P2O5, and K2O, respectively. The N:P2O5:K2O ratio of 28:5:1 is highly unbalanced, due to the very high N application (282 kg N ha-1) compared to the very small K application (10 kg K2O ha-1). In order to evaluate the effect of potassium in a typical crop rotation performed in districts of Punjab, IPI has initiated research and extension activities at the KVK Bahowal, Directorate of Extension of Punjab Agriculture University. The effect of K was demonstrated in farmers' fields in 5 districts on a typical pea-sunflower-maize crop rotation, grown on sandy loam soil. This project has a specific extension character and includes demonstration plots, farmers' field days, and literature in the local language. Both scientific and extension activities were possible in these experiments.

Soybean is grown on about 4.5 million ha in the State of Madhya Pradesh and production accounts for 59% of India's total. In 2004, the Secretary of Agriculture of the State declared that in 8 districts 100,000 ha of soybean had been completely damaged by pests and insects. Total area affected was almost 1 million ha, about 25% of the total area growing soybean in the State.

Often better plant nutrition decreases the susceptibility of crops to attacks by insects and diseases, and this reduces the need for pesticides and insecticides. Results from various experiments performed by IPI and by IRRI show that applying K reduces the damage caused by insects and disease. The effect of potash application on soybean was demonstrated in an IPI experiment in Indore, Madhya Pradesh through the project "Studies on role of potassium nutrition in balanced fertilization of Soybean-Wheat cropping system". One of the major effects for potash application was consistent reduction of infestation and incidence of various insects and disease.

A reduction of 50% to 75% of the damage was observed in farmers' fields, resulting in large savings of pesticides and insecticides. In addition, potash application increased nodule number and dry weight (60% and 100% respectively) and consequently the yield (35%). Perrenoud reviewed almost 2450 literature references on this subject and concluded that the use of K decreased the incidence of fungal diseases in 70%

of cases. The corresponding decrease of other pests was bacteria 69%, insects and mites 63%, and viruses 41%. Simultaneously, K increased the yield of plants infested with fungal diseases by 42%, with bacteria by 57%, with insects and mites by 36%, and with viruses by 78%. Kafkafi et al. recently reviewed the role of both K and chloride on the suppression of diseases and stresses in plants. Potassium may exert its greatest effect on disease through specific metabolic functions that alter the compatibility relationship of the host parasite environment. A number of possible mechanisms may be involved. These include: (i) enhanced host tolerance due to increased water potential that restricts infection by pathogens and, in consequence, plants are better able to withstand disease; (ii) suppression inhibition of pathogens through lower tissue which decreases crop susceptibility nitrification inhibition and to increased soil NH4 + and NH4 + uptake, resulting in rhizosphere acidification.

Better nutrient management, which involved reduced and split N application, along with increased P and K application, reduced the intensity of disease by 50% and increased yield by 12.5%. These results from the Site Specific Nutrient Management project in the Philippines demonstrate the positive effect of nutrient management on plant health.

The economics of balanced fertilization The "Reaching Towards Optimal Productivity" workgroup of the Irrigated Rice Research Consortium has been instrumental in the development, evaluation, and promotion of site specific nutrient management as an approach for increasing the profit of Asian rice farmers through more efficient use of plant nutrients. It operates through partnerships with the national agricultural research and extension systems in Bangladesh, China, India, Indonesia, Myanmar, Philippines, Thailand, and Vietnam.

In 2005, RTOP activities were incorporated into the new "Productivity and Sustainability" workgroup of Phase III of the IRRC. The project demonstrates the importance of N management through the use of the Leaf Color Chart (LCC) in increasing N use efficiency and yields, and consequently larger P and K requirements. Potassium fertilization recommendations are calculated through SSNM plots on farmers' fields, taking into account also the amount of straw recycled back to the field.

The economics of SSNM have been analyzed for recent years. Table 5 shows the increased net profit gained from using the SSNM approach. Farmers in Southern India increased their net profit by 47%, while those in Southern Vietnam by only 4.25%. This calculation does not take into account additional benefits, even though not directly related to the farmers, of smaller N losses to the environment through emissions to the atmosphere and leaching.

The RTOP workgroup is supported also by IFA, IPI, and PPI. Educational and extension activities are performed both at the scientific level and by meetings at the field level. Recommended K levels set by the local extension service) match the latest findings of SSNM in the Old Delta in Southern India, reflecting the need to promote these to farmers. However, in the New Delta, the higher K rates recommended by SSNM need to be addressed at research, extension, and farmers levels to be brought into practice to benefit farmers.

Conclusions

Long-term negative K balances, mainly caused by insufficient K fertilization and limited use of crop residues required for increased yields, cause deterioration of soil fertility that leads to stagnating and decreased production. Common reasons for inadequate K use are the farmers' lack of knowledge, and frequently of their advisors, as well as socio-economical factors. The constant shift from staple low cost crops to high value horticultural crops is a major driver in correcting unbalanced fertilization.

7

Increasing Crop Production: Biological Processes

The designations employed and the presentation of material in this information product do not imply the expression of any opinion whatsoever on the part of the Food and Agriculture Organization of the United Nations (FAO) concerning the legal or development status of any country, territory, city or area or of its authorities, or concerning the delimitation of its frontiers or boundaries. The mention of specific companies or products of manufacturers, whether or not these have been patented, does not imply that these have been endorsed or recommended by FAOin preference to others of a similar nature that are not mentioned. With global population expected to exceed 9 billion by 2050, agricultural production Would need to groWglobally by 70 percent over the same period to feed this population. This need to feed more people puts greater pressure on crop production and the resource base upon which it depends. this is exacerbated by the additional pressures of coping with an increasingly degraded environment, uncertainties arising from climate change and other stressors such as increasing urbanization and volatile food prices.

Further complicating this situation is that the global community must meet this increasing food demand in a world where ecosystem resilience is compromised, and land resources available for agricultural expansion are limited.

With land scarcity, crop production intensification rather than area expansion becomes the primary option available. Well-managed ecosystems are essential for ensuring a healthy resource base on which to intensify sustainably, to ensure that enough food is produced from now until 2050 and beyond.

farming practices are shifting away from heavy dependency on non-renewable inputs and chemical-based intensification, such as the use of pesticides. instead, they are moving towards other forms of intensification, relying on natural biological processes and biodiversity to increase the productivity of agroecosystems.

The underpinning scientific and biological principles for improving soil health, managing pollination or controlling pest populations - incorporated in farming practices - show that yields can be increased through the sustainable management of ecosystems.

Here, the role of farmers as custodians of biodiversity and as ecosystem managers is essential. At local levels, farming practices, approaches or technologies based on the management of biological processes that provide essential ecosystem goods and services, can be applied to produce higher crop yields and optimize input use while maintaining or enhancing ecosystem health. Arange of options exist for good farm management practices, approaches and technologies that are based on biological processes. Examples include: conservation agriculture; integrated plant nutrient management; integrated pest management; and pollination management. These farm management practices are being increasingly used to achieve sustainable crop production intensification which has a key role in feeding the world, today and in the future.

To increase future food production, crop production will need to adapt to and mitigate climate change. The negative effects of climate change on productivity, which are already being felt by the agriculture sector today, can only be addressed through better understanding of the biological processes involved in farm management practices. In this regard, ecosystem management must incorporate measures of resilience and risk mitigation into agriculture elements that are increasingly relevant under changing climates.

While rice production was boosted through irrigation, seeds of new varieties and fertilizer during the 1970s the so-called "green revolution", that production was threatened in the 1980s by large scale insect pest outbreaks, especially of the rice brown planthopper. resistant rice varieties were bred by researchers and distributed by national seed systems, but as pest populations evolved they often lost their effectiveness, and insect outbreaks continued to spread, damaging rice severely or even killing plants.

Bold policy reforms in the 1990s to remove insecticide subsidies, and support for widespread farmer education through Farmer Field Schools and similar campaigns, were combined to reduce insecticide use and stop the pest outbreaks. In the Philippines, between 1996 and 2007, national rice production increased by 60 percent and rice yield per hectare increased by 12 percent. During this period numbers of both insecticide applications and total active ingredients used were reduced by more than 70 percent.

The Perspective of Biological Processes

Elsewhere these trends have been sustained over several decades. For instance, in Indonesia the cost of insecticides used on rice dropped by over 75 percent while national rice production grew by more than 25 percent between 1986, when the national IPMpolicy was first declared, and 2001. In India, from 1994 to 2002 total food grain production rose by over 20 percent while tons of pesticides used fell by over 35 percent. Some predators attack the eggs of the BPH, following the trail left by pregnant females when they lay their eggs in the stem of the rice plant, and sucking out each egg in a row along the stem. Some predators live only on the surface of fresh water, such as in ponds, streams, and rice paddies. They attack the newly hatched young BPHthat fall onto the water every day. Predatory spiders can kill and eat over 20 BPHevery day, in order to mature their own eggs and produce more young predators. These predators, and many more like them, fulfil the ecosystem function of naturally occurring biological pest control in annual crop systems like rice. Their ecosystem function grows or shrinks as the predators multiply or leave to other fields in their search for larger populations of the pests. Their ecosystem function renews itself through the arrival and reproduction of predators in rice paddies, which depends on their food source: the pests.

By enhancing this ecosystem function, by making the rice field ecosystem healthier, more ecosystem services are provided in this case, pest control. Of course there are situations where the predator populations are not able to respond in time, such as after massive floods or extended drought, but the decision to apply insecticides should be made in each rice paddy based on the numbers of predators as well as the crop condition and the numbers of pests.

Making these informed decisions, optimizing and adapting management on a field-to-field basis, means that farmers must build their own knowledge systems using up-to-date ecological concepts, like predation.

FAOhas worked in the field with many national agricultural systems, research, extension, academic, Non-Governmental Organizations, and farmers' community organizations to provide these ecological concepts to millions of rice farmers in hundreds of thousands of Farmer Field Schools.

The absence of pollination can cause significant declines in *quantity* of produce, but evidence shows that absence of pollination also has a negative effect on the *quality* of fruits and seed set. The table on the next page shows crops that can experience declines in production – by up to 90 percent if they lack pollination.

Pollination management practices can also be applied to mitigate climate change. Many good farming practices that sustain the ability of agroecosystems to deliver ecosystem services involve measures to increase ground cover and crop-associated biodiversity. Hence, measures to promote pollinators include providing more non-crop flowering resources in fields, such as cover crops, strip crops or hedgerows.

Phosphorus (P): a major plant nutrient

Pused as a fertilizer is a finite resource, mainly obtained through mining (i.e. rock phosphate). It is one of the three major elements for plant nutrition and an essential component for the functioning and development of plants. In the soil it can be easily immobilized, making it inaccessible to plant roots in most tropical soils, making it a limiting factor for crop production. It is important to find ways to mobilize Pfrom soils and make it available to plants. This can be achieved through the promotion of *mycorrhiza* and increased associated biological activity in the soil-root system.

> *Mycorrhiza* fungus forms a symbiotic association with the roots of plants. It can either penetrate the root cells (endomycorrhiza) or not (ectomycorrhiza), and promotes root growth and extends the root system, supplying plants with P.

> *Mycorrhiza produces organic acids, stabilizes pH, and mobilizes immobile P, including in high pH soils.*

Nutrient pumps: deep roots help achieve nutrient balance

Soils rich in organic matter have a pool of well-balanced nutrients that contribute to crop growth and plant development. Such soils avoid the problems that result from unbalanced plant nutrition such as lower fertilizer use efficiency and reduced crop quality.

> Balanced nutrient supply from organic matter pool is important for optimal plant growth and development.

> Deep rooting crops act as nutrient pumps with their decaying crop residues.

Nitrogen (N): a major building block for protein certain bacteria convert atmospheric nitrogen into organic nitrogenous compounds which provide nutrition for plant growth and for soil microorganisms. > there are symbiotic n-fixing bacteria, such as *rhizobia* which are found in root nodules of legumes including pulses, oil seeds, trees and shrubs, and pasture legumes there are free living n-fixing bacteria such as *azotobactor* and *Beijerinkia* that live in the soil and root rhyzosphere, the area of soil surrounding the roots of plants.these bacteria convert atmospheric nitrogen (n2) into organic nitrogenous compounds which provide nutrition for plant growth and for soil microorganisms.nitrogen-fixing root nodules of legumes.

Biological Nitrogen Fixation

in agricultural systems, some types of microbes can achieve biological nitrogen fixation (Bnf) as free-living organisms: heterotrophic and autotrophic bacteria and cyanobacteria. other micro-organisms can only fix nitrogen through a symbiosis with plants, mainly legume species. in agricultural areas, about 80 percent of Bnf is achieved by such a symbiotic association, between the legumes and the nodule bacteria, the *rhizobia*.

Nitrogen transfer to other crops or forages

Nitrogen fixed by legumes is harvested in the crop and partly transferred to subsequent crops increasing their yields. For instance, in forage legume/grass mixtures, nitrogen is transferred from legume to grass (e.g. 13 to 34 percent of fixed N). In cutting meadows, Nis exported with silage or hay and ingested by animals. About 70–95 percent of this nitrogen is excreted by animals and the manure can then be recycled by spreading on arable land.

Impact of legumes on natural resources

The direct environmental cost associated with legume-based systems is marginally lower than that of Nfertilized-based systems. The risk of nitrate leaching depends very much on farming practices and is not always lower in legume-based systems. N2Oemissions seem to be comparable in both systems. However, synthesis of chemical fertilizer requires large amounts of fossil energy. By contrast BNFis based on solar energy and does not emit CO2 into the atmosphere.

The introduction of legumes (legume cover crops, grass/legume pastures, legume-based fallow or even annual legume crops) in crop rotations has proven to reduce weed infestation, disease and pest attacks.

Legume-based cropping systems contribute to maintaining biodiversity, especially of pollinators, other arthropods, soil life in general, and many of the bird and mammal species that are able to live in agricultural landscapes.

Importance of legumes for sustainable agriculture

In the context of increasing prices of fossil fuels and mineral Nfertilizers, a progressive shift from Nfertilizers to N-fixing legumes would seem to be highly desirable. Current BNFby crop legumes is estimated globally at about 20–22 million tonnes of Neach year. There is potential to harness more if the relevant biological processes are promoted within legume-based production systems.

Another element of biological tillage is the introduction of crops including trees and shrubs with deep penetrating tap-roots. Some of these "pioneer" crops such as lupine, jack-beans or radish can break subsoil compactions, if for example, planted in the crop rotation or in intercrop association as green manure cover crops.

The problem is that most agricultural soils no longer provide a suitable living environment for the micro-organisms that are so critical to these processes. Even when they are used – those such as *rhizobia* or even *mycorrhiza* may become inoculants for specific crops – they do not flourish in farming systems that rely on mechanical tillage because tillage stirs up the soil and creates a major interruption in the soil habitat which is not tolerated by most organisms that normally live in undisturbed soil.

8

The Role of Micronutrients in Crop Production and Human Health

The soils in Pakistan across 22 Mha cultivated area are predominantly alluvial and loessal, alkaline in pH, calcareous and low in organic matter. These factors are mainly responsible for nutrient fixation in soil and low availability to plants. Zinc deficiency in Pakistan was the first micronutrient disorder recognised in early 1970s as a cause of *hadda* disease in rice. After identification of Zn deficiency, extensive research has been carried out during last four decades on micronutrient deficiencies in soils and their drastic effects on crops. Subsequently, field-scale deficiencies of zinc boron and iron have been established in many field and horticultural crops. The most widespread deficiency is of Zn as 70 % of the soils of Pakistan are Zn deficient and observed in rice, wheat, cotton, maize, sunflower, sugarcane, brassica, potato and in many other crops along with citrus and deciduous fruits. Boron deficiency is another major nutritional disorder which severely affects rice, cotton, wheat, sugarbeet, peanut, citrus and deciduous fruits. The third field-scale disorder is Fe chlorosis which has been exhibited in peanut, chickpea, cotton, citrus, ornamentals and many tree species. Copper and manganese deficiencies are of localized occurrence.

The mineral elements like Zn, Fe and Cu are as crucial for human health as organic compounds such as carbohydrates, fats, protein and vitamins. The daily dietary intake of young adult ranges from 10-60 mg for Fe, 2-3 mg for Cu and 15 mg for Zn. Intake less than these values can cause slow physiological processes. These micronutrients deficiencies in soil are not only hampering the crop productivity but also are deteriorating produce quality. High consumption of cereal based foods with low contents of micronutrients is causing health hazards in humans. The contents of micronutrients in food can be elevated either by supplementation, fortification or by agricultural strategies i.e., biofortification and application of micronutrients containing fertilizers.

Food fortification and supplementation are too expensive, not practical to be applied on large scale and not easily accessible to poor masses. The development of micronutrient efficient genotypes can be a successive tool to overcome the micronutrient disorders in soil and for improvement in human health. However, the harvesting of micronutrient enriched grains from field would mine out more micronutrients. The cultivation of these genotypes can be integrated with the application of micronutrients containing fertilizers. Addition of such fertilizers will not only correct the deficiencies but also improve the fruit size and quality of crops. In general, 2-5 kg Zn ha-1 may be adequate for improved crop production, however, soil applied Fe is generally ineffective except for Fe-sequestrine. Repeated sprays of Ferrous sulphate (FeSO4) or chelated Fe cure the chlorosis and improve the quality of food stuff. However, despite being highly cost effective, currently micronutrient use is negligible.

Introduction

The elements essential for plants are C, H, O, N, P, K, Ca, Mg, S, Fe, Cu, B, Mn, Mo, Zn, Cl. Out of these 16 elements, 9 essential elements have been classified as "macronutrients" as these are required in relatively large amount by the plants. These elements include C, H, O, N, P, K, Ca, Mg, S. The remaining of the elementsare called "trace elements". The group of essential elements includes both macro and trace elements. Essential trace elements are often called "micronutrients" because they are required in small, but in critical concentrations by living organisms. Out of 80 million hectare geographical area of Pakistan, 22 Mha are cultivated. The cultivated soils of the country have derived from alluvium and loess, and are low in organic matter and many essential nutrients. The deficiency of Zn, Fe and Cu is the common feature of these soils. Being arid to semi arid area, about 75% of cultivated area is irrigated while the rest is rain-fed. The major cropping systems in the country are cotton- wheat, rice-wheat and mixed cropping like maize based and sugarcane based systems. Popular crops in rain-fed area are wheat, sorghum, peanut, chickpea etc. Usually two crops in a year is the normal routine unless moisture is a serious problem. As a matter of fact whole crop produce is removed from the field, hardly any crop residue is recycled back into the soil. In addition abundant soil moisture particularly during monsoon season may cause micronutrient leaching beyond the root zone while the soil surface due to dry spell may also retard the root absorption of micronutrients. During the era of "Green

Revolution" the high yielding crop varieties were introduced and their higher demand for nutrients also contributed to increased amount of micronutrients mining which lead to their deficiencies. Unfortunately, fertilizer application practice in Pakistan is predominantly in favour of nitrogen (N) and phosphorus (P) only, whereas potassium (K) use is limited to a few high K requiring crops like sugarcane and potatoes. Many introduced crop varieties are more susceptible to micronutrient deficiencies than landraces.

According to a survey about 70% of the soils used for growing crops in Pakistan have low levels of available Zn (Rashid, 1996). Zinc deficiency in plants does not only reduce the yield but also the nutritional quality of grains. Hence soil conditions and agronomic practices are conducive to the incidence of micronutrient deficiencies in plants. The production of low micronutrient stuff has created concern about micronutrient-deficiency related health hazards especially in poor masses of society in developing countries of the world. It is imperative to initiate studies on such global problems with due attention. This paper will review the role of micronutrients in crop production and human health.

Micronutrient deficiencies: Deficiency of micronutrient in soil and plants is a global nutritional problem and is prevalent in many countries with different magnitude of severity. The identification of biological role of Zn by Raulin who observed that common bread mold did not grow in the absence of Zn. This observation introduced a new area for research in crops, and in 1914 first demonstration of Zn deficiency in plants was made by Mazé while the first identification of Zn deficiency in field conditions was reported by in the deciduous orchards of California. Deficiency of other micronutrient was established in the same era. The countries affected by micronutrient deficiency include USA, Australia, Turkey, India, Pakistan and other countries.

In Pakistan the first ever micronutrient deficiency was observed by Yashida & Tanaka who established that the cause of *Hadda* disease of rice in the Punjab was Zn deficiency. Field scale Zn deficiency in rice in Punjab was established in 1970. During 1980, micronutrient deficiencies were recognized in a wide range of soils, crops and fruits in NWFP, Punjab, Balochistan, Sindh and Azad Jammu and Kashmir. A wide spread deficiency of Zn, Fe and B in rainfed soils and crops of Pothowar plateau was also established in the same period.

Diagnosis of micronutrients deficiencies - plant deficiency symptoms: As the micronutrient deficient plants may exhibit characteristic symptoms, plant symptoms can be useful indicator of micronutrient deficiencies. The most common symptoms of Zn deficiency include stunted growth, shortened internodes and petioles and small malformed leaves which result in "rosette" symptom in young growth of dicotyledons and "fan shaped" stem in monocotyledons. Deficiency symptoms of Cu are dieback of stems and twigs, yellowing of leaves, stunted growth and pale green leaves that wither easily. In case of iron deficiency chlorosis of young leaves is peculiar in many crops and fruit plants. Other micronutrients have also characteristics symptoms by which their deficiencies can be identified in plants.

Soil testing: It is practical and most widely used technique for predicting micronutrients deficiencies in crops. An ideal soil test is one which is rapid, reproducible and correlates reliably with responses in plant yield, plant specific nutrient concentration or uptake of that nutrient. However, soil test levels at which micronutrient deficiency in plant can occur may vary to some extent according to soil type and crop species. Soil samples for the analysis can be taken at any time of the year but care is needed to ensure that a representative sample has been taken over the full area of the field. It is also important to avoid contamination of the soil samples by contact with metal equipment. The soil tests most widely used around the world include AB-DTPA and DTPA. These are multielement soil tests for alkaline soils and effective as conventional micronutrient tests for Cu, Fe, Zn and Mn. Generalized micronutrient soil test interpretation criteria for determining micronutrient deficiencies in Pakistan.

Plant analysis: An alternative to soil testing is to analyse samples of leaves or grain to determine the micronutrient status of both crop and soil on which it is growing. However, it is not often possible to rectify the problem to prevent the losses in the existing crop, but once diagnosed, the deficiency can be treated for future crops in time to prevent further losses of yield. Leaf sampling practices vary with regard to which leaves are sampled and this is the result of local experience. However, in all cases, after sampling the leaves need to be thoroughly washed with distilled water and dried before grinding for analysis, taking care to avoid contact of the sample with external sources of micronutrients at all stages. Critical or threshold concentrations in leaf dry matter will also vary according to the species of plant and the position of the leaves on the plant. In general, critical leaf values range from 15 mg Zn kg-1 in rice, 20 mg Zn kg-1 in wheat, and 22 mg Zn kg-1 in maize and groundnut.

Factors affecting micronutrient bioavailability: Bioavailability of all four metallic micronutrients is significantly affected by soil pH, decreasing with increasing soil pH. Solubility of Fe decreases a thousand fold for each unit increase in soil pH in the range 4 to 9 and consequently, most Fe deficiencies occur on calcareous soils. The activity (consequent bioavailability) of Mn, Cu and Zn decreases 100-fold for each unit increase in soil pH. Amounts of exchangeable metals in soil are related to their concentrations in soil solutions, so soil pH affects exchangeable Fe, Mn, Cu and Zn similarly.

Reactions with soil organic matter significantly affect the bioavailability of these metallic micronutrients. Copper reacts with SOM to form very stable complexes with carboxylic and phenolic groups. Due to these stable complexes Cu deficiencies are often associated with organic soils. Reactions of Zn with SOM are also important in providing bioavailable Zn, but the strength of these bonds is not as strong as with Cu.

There are many other factors like calcium carbonate contents, clay contents, concentrations of other nutrients, salt affected soils and water logging which can affect the bioavailability of micronutrients to plants.

Soil types associated with widespread micronutrient deficiencies in crops: Although it is recognised that micronutrients deficiencies in crops can be found on many types of soils in the different bio - climatic zones of the world, there are a relatively small number of widely occurring types of soil which are more frequently associated with micronutrient deficiencies than any other. These are:

1. Calcareous soils
2. Organic soils
3. Sandy soils
4. Saline and Sodic (salt- affected) soils
5. Vertisols,
6. Gleysols poorly drained waterlogged soils.

Susceptibility of crops to zinc deficiency: All crops are susceptible to zinc deficiency, but species differ considerably in their ability to tolerate low levels of zinc supply. The relative susceptibilities of different crop species to zinc deficiency.

However, even though wheat has a relatively low susceptibility, it is still affected by deficiency in many parts of the world where the available zinc status of soils is very low. Much of the land in Asia and the Near East and Australia used for wheat production has either calcareous or sandy soils with very low zinc supply capacities and this causes yield losses of 20% or more over vast areas. Paddy rice production on flooded soils is also very prone to zinc deficiency and it is estimated that up to 50% of all paddy rice production could be affected by zinc deficiency.

Improving crop yield and quality with micronutrients: Micronutrient deficiency can greatly disturb plant yield and quality, and the health of domestic animals and humans. Extensive research on the effects of micronutrient fertilizers on crop yield and quality has been conducted during the past decade. Results of a broad-based study conducted in 815 irrigated wheat growing regions of Iran to evaluate the effect of micronutrients showed an increase of 4 to 11% in wheat grain yield by the addition of each micronutrient or a combination of Fe + Zn + Cu + B to NPK fertilizer increased grain yield.

Appreciable crop yield increases under local conditions have also been observed in a number of crops at the farmers' fields. Average yield increases with Zn application are 22% in potato and sunflower, 18% in maize, 13% in wheat, 12% in rice and 8% in sugarcane. Average yield increases with B have been depicted from 7% to 21% in different crops. In Pakistan, the peanut, potato and chickpea are severely affected by Fe deficiency and the yield increased recorded by the use of Fe averaged as 30% for peanut, 16% for potato and 15% for chickpea. Inorganic Fe salts except Sequestrene are generally ineffective in soil application. However, repeated foliar sprays of FeSO4 or chelated Fe cure the chlorosis.

Mineral nutrient reserves in seed must also be adequate to sustain plant growth until root system takes over the nutrient supply function. During early establishment phase, the mineral nutrients are partly supplied by the soil. Therefore, information on mineral nutrient reserves in seed should be perfect from agricultural point of view and human requirements as well. It could provide an insight into these genotypes, which are high mineral element accumulators, and can best be utilized for human consumption as well as agricultural production. In the absence of systematic data it would be very difficult to determine the adequacy of our diet with respect to minerals.

The seed of a number of wheat genotypes was analysed for different micronutrients concentrations and it was found that none of these genotypes fulfil the quality standards set by the Harvest Plus. According to Harvest Plus, for improved micronutrient nutrition of humans, cereals grains should contain 50 to 60 mg kg-1 Zn and similar amount of Fe. This situation is very alarming and there is a dire need for an alternative and a rapid approach to improve mineral nutrient concentrations in cereals.

Human health: Micronutrient malnutrition, the so-called hidden hunger, affects more than one-half of the world's population, especially women and preschool children in developing countries. The role of micronutrients such as vitamin A, iodine, iron and zinc in human nutrition has increasingly been recognized over the last decade. This has led to a change of paradigms in nutrition research and policy, away from the 'traditional' protein-energy-malnutrition focus. The physiological impacts of micronutrients are complex, relating to many bodily functions. Zinc deficiency has serious consequences for human health including: impairment of the immune system and as a result, increased prevalence of childhood infections, such as diarrhoea and pneumonia; impaired growth and development of infants, children and adolescents; impaired maternal health and pregnancy outcome. Not least the impact of zinc deficiency on immune system defects is of interest in South Asia where as much as

95% of the population is at risk, due to poverty and rice-pulse diets. Trials conducted in several countries indicate that duration and severity of major baby-killers such as diarrhoea and pneumonia can be reduced by 30-50 % by supplying adequate amounts of vitamin A and zinc. In developing countries, zinc deficiency ranks 5th among the leading 10 risk factors. Even on a global scale, taking developed and developing countries together, zinc deficiency ranks 11th out of the 20 leading risk factors. WHO attributes 800,000 deaths worldwide each year to zinc deficiency and over 28 million healthy life years lost. It is estimated that zinc deficiency affects one-third of the world's population, with estimates ranging from 4 to 73% according to region and it is 5th leading risk factor alongwith the Fe deficiency which is at 6th position globally.

Pakistan has also been affected by the malnutrition of both these elements. Iron and Zn deficiencies are extremely high in pregnant/lactating women as well as in very young children. This confirms the high levels of anaemia and other Zn related diseases in these groups. It has been estimated that extent of Zn deficiency in population ranges from 36 to 49% and that of Fe deficiency from 45 to 65%. There is a dire need for a rapid approach to improve mineral nutrient concentrations in cereals. Different strategies listed below can be helpful in enhancing the micronutrient densities in staple foods.

Supplementation: Providing Zn or other micronutrients in tablets, syrups etc., to vulnerable groups through health care is possible, but may not be a practical solution in socially or geographically marginal populations.

Food fortification: The addition of nutrients to commonly eaten foods, beverages or condiments. It has played a major role in eliminating micronutrient deficiencies in industrialized countries. Infant formulas, infant cereals and ready-to-eat breakfast cereals are often fortified with Zn. Mexico is presently conducting a national, voluntary zinc fortification program, where Zn and other micronutrients are added to wheat and corn flours used for preparing bread and tortilla.

Fortification of wheat flour with Fe is an option which also being carried out at NIFA, Peshawar in Pakistan. In Thailand, Zn and Fe enriched noodles are being marketed. With regards to Zn supplies to the poorer parts of the population in South Asia, there has not yet been identified a good food vector. Despite past progress in controlling micronutrient deficiencies through supplementation and food fortification, new approaches are needed to expand the research of food-based interventions possibly through agricultural strategies.

Biofortification: Biofortification, a new approach that relies on conventional plant breeding and modern biotechnology to increase the micronutrient density of staple crops, holds great promise for improving the nutritional status and health of poor populations in both rural and urban areas of the developing world. Biofortification provides a sustainable solution to Fe and Zn deficiencies in food around the world as it is the process of enriching the nutrient contents of staple crops.

Biofortification of staple food crops with micronutrients by either breeding for higher uptake efficiency or fertilization can be an effective strategy to address widespread dietary deficiency in human populations. The lack of micronutrients such as Fe and Zn is a widespread nutrition and health problem in developing countries. Reports have highlighted the current strategies for the biofortification of crops, including mineral fertilization, conventional breeding and transgenic approaches. Any approach which could increase root growth and result in a high transfer of Fe and Zn from the soil to the plant is crucial for biofortification.

Genotypic differences in micronutrient use efficiency: Micronutrient efficiency is the ability of a crop to grow and yield well when the availability of the micronutrient is low. Field and growth room screening has shown significant genetic variation in Zn and manganese efficiency in winter cereals, which indicates that selection for improved micronutrient efficiency is possible.

When grown on soils with low micronutrient availability due to either chemical or biological fixation, or spatial or temporal unavailability, micronutrient-efficient genotypes have a greater yield in comparison to inefficient ones, even when fertilized with smaller amounts of fertilizers or less frequently. Generally, micronutrient-efficient genotypes are capable of increasing available soil micronutrient pools through changing chemical and microbiological properties of the rhizosphere as well as by growing thinner and longer roots and having more efficient uptake and transport systems. For Zn-efficient genotypes, more efficient utilization of Zn in tissue also contributes to overall Zn efficiency. Understanding micronutrient efficiency mechanisms is important for designing suitable screening techniques for breeding micronutrient-efficient genotypes. Growing micronutrient-efficient genotypes contributes to environmentally-benign agriculture by lowering the input of chemicals and energy.

These genotypes also offer a potential for producing grain for human consumption with higher concentration of Fe, Zn and Cu, the three micronutrients that about a third of the world population is deficient. Such studies have been conducted in Pakistan with many domestic and exotic wheat genotypes for Zn efficiency which show that these genotypes have different Zn efficiencies which can be exploited for biofortification strategies.

Breeding strategy is however, a long term process requiring different types of efforts and resources and it is uncertain whether the breeding strategy will work or not after these long term efforts over many years and huge investments. Apart from these constraints, harvesting of micronutrient-enriched grains from the field through biofortified genotypes can remove more these from land and cause rapid depletion of available soil micronutrients, further aggravating deficiencies in soil. A successful breeding program for bio-fortifying cereals is very much dependent on the amount of plant available micronutrients in the soil.

Fertilizer strategies: Micronutrient deficiency is widespread in many Asian countries including Pakistan due to the calcareous nature of soils, high pH, low organic matter, salt stress, continuous drought, high bicarbonate content in irrigation water, and imbalanced application of fertilizers. Some of the adverse effects of micronutrient deficiency-induced stress in plants include low crop yield and quality, imperfect plant morphological structure (such as fewer xylem vessels of small size), widespread infestation of various diseases and pests, low activation of phytosiderophores, and lower fertilizer use efficiency. The absence of micronutrient fertilizers results in inadequate absorption of trace elements by plants, which causes substantial yield losses in different crops and forages, and eventually results in poor health for domestic animals and humans. Calcareous soil research results of the last decade show that at the present time, among micronutrients, Zn deficiency is the most detrimental to effect crop yield. Other important micronutrients that increase crop yield (most to least effect) are Fe, B, Mn, Cu, and Mo. In the case of calcareous soils, the conventional notion that micronutrients increase crop yield by 15-30% is an underestimated range. In fact, in some cases, especially with inefficient cultivars such as durum wheat, micronutrients can increase grain yield up to 50%, as well as increase macronutrient use efficiency. By supplying plants with micronutrients, either through soil application, foliar spray, or seed treatment, increased yield and higher quality, as well as macronutrient use efficiency, could be achieved.

The application of micronutrient fertilizers not only increase the yield of the crop but also increase the density of nutrients in the grain which is now prerequisite for the human health. Adding regular fertilizer to soil for crop production can be a better strategy along with the biofortification as it is simple, requires less efforts and provides substantial benefits as mentioned above. In our local soil conditions, following rates of micronutrients application have been recommended for better harvest.

Conclusion

Micronutrients nutrition of crops has immense economic importance since an adequate supply of micronutrients can help to ensure that optimum yields are obtained with the given inputs of other crop requirements. It is essential that the available micronutrients status of arable soils is checked on a regular basis to ensure that easily preventable deficiency is not adversely affecting crop productivity and quality. As the deficiency of Zn is widespread in our country, the farmers and agronomists need to always think about Zn.

9

Pesticides: A Contribution to Agriculture and Nutrition

This a pleasure for me to address myself to the subject of pesticides in relation to nutrition, for it is in this area that pesticides make their great contribution to our health as a nation and to the world's health. I think it is important, first, to attempt to bring the subject of nutrition and food supply somewhat into focus. I am certain that it is trite for me to state that the United States is one of the most abundantly fed nations of the world. Yet, because it is so commonplace, we perhaps fail at times to recognize that our housewives have access to the greatest variety of foodstuffs ever made available to a general population of any country. Their daily choices in foods exceed those of the royalty of yesteryear, thanks to the unprecedented strides in the production, processing, distribution, marketing, and conservation of food we have made, especially, during the last three decades.

Those of us who were reared in rural America remember the general store, with its cracker barrel-and, if in the South, its salt pork and molasses-its overalls, and a handful of tins, in which the housewife, if she were fortunate in her home canning, might preserve some of her garden tomatoes, using sealing wax to tack down the lids. These would help carry the family over the winter, and, as we now recognize, help to prevent scurvy. Contrast to this the modem- day supermarkets, with their thousands of foods items, and with the complete, or near complete disappearance of seasonal foods, seasonal fruits, seasonal vegetables, and indeed, even seasonal meats-except for those which cater to our appetites in relation to particular seasonal holidays and festivities! We have experienced in this century a revolution in foods in the technically developed countries of North America and Western Europe, and in Australia and some other areas. This enviable achievement has been attained by the application and exploitation of science to agriculture and to food technology.

It has been accompanied by the virtual disappearance from the United States of all the major deficiency diseases. We have seen the disappearance of pellagra. This disease was prevalent not only in the South, but in the Corn Belt; indeed, it was in Illinois, in 1912, that there was established what was to become a very famous commission for the study of pellagra in the state. It was that commission, incidentally, which concluded that pellagra was an infectious disease.

We have seen the disappearance, or near disappearance, of endemic goiter, protein malnutrition, vitamin A deficiency riboflavin deficiency, and rickets- all now are rarities, rather than major health problems. The average adult stature in our country has constantly increased; today, we are taller than ever before. We now have the lowest death rate and the longest life expectancy in our history; we are living long enough to experience an increase in the diseases of old age, that is, the degenerative diseases, including cancer and cardiovasiscular disease. It is the importance of these diseases within an aged population, for which at the same time there is protection from the infectious diseases and other causes of death-including the deficiency states I have just mentioned-that has focused public attention on them. The absence of definitive understanding of the pathogenesis and the etiology of some of these diseases, coupled with the recognition of their toll among our aged population, creates the fear and anxiety of ignorance. Thus, there is a tendency among many persons in our population to blame one or another new development for these diseases- often without rationale or logic. These prophets of doom, with their pat answers to problems, overlook or ignore the true state of the nation's health. During this century there also has occurred a social revolution, industrialization and urbanization, coupled with an "off the farm" movement. It seems highly improbable that this trend will reverse itself. Increased efficiency of farm production has maintained our food supply, despite this decrease in proportion of the population engaged in farm operations; in 1940, it was estimated that the labor of one farmer produced food and fiber sufficient for about 11 persons; today he provides enough for from 26 to 29 individuals. One may illustrate these changes on the farm in another way: with 30 per cent less farm employment, and 43 million more people in the nation than in 1940, there is more raw material produced per capita of the population today.

A part of these revolutions has been the intense, concentrated, scientific form of agricultural crop management. This makes for efficiency, but at the same time makes crop lands more susceptible to disastrous losses due to unexpected or uncontrolled epidemics of plant diseases, or invasion by uncontrolled animal pests. This situation is not unlike that which arises in the human population as it becomes urbanized with greater concentration, there occurs a greater opportunity for spread of disease, and, as a result, there is a greater need for control and preventive measures.

The United States produces food commodities in excess of what we can presently consume. This excess constitutes our so-called farm surplus. It is argued by many that the existence of this farm surplus means that we can-and even should-take measures to reverse the trends which I have just described. Such measures are advocated as a return to less sophisticated methods of agriculture or food processing than we now practice. Indeed, many hold that the present state of affairs is unhealthy, and is, or may be, causing us to die of the "diseases of our aging population," those diseases which affect particularly the aged, which I have just mentioned. They ignore the fact that the present sophisticated food supply methods in fact are permitting us to remain alive long enough to become victims of these diseases. These people cite our current farm surpluses as evidence that any decrease in production would not matter and might even be beneficial. They ignore the usefulness of a food reserve to us, and to less-well-fed populations elsewhere. They do not include in their own plans the feeding of tomorrow's children.

I fear that these well intentioned people more often than not are unrealistically narrow in their understanding either of the present or of the future, and, though at times they are painfully anxious in their ignorance, they are yet missionary in their zeal to save this nation from its present state of good health.

Our population is reproducing vigorously and, since babies now live longer, we are growing in numbers. The size of this growth in the population, in relation to agricultural production, has been admirably summarized by a number of persons. I should like to quote from one of them, Dr. George McNew: "What will be the needs of this nation a decade from now? By 1975 we can expect to have a population of about 210,000,000 people since our net rate of increase is approximately three million persons per year. To supply these people adequately we need to add productivity equivalent to about six million acres per year. There simply are not to be found some 60 million acres each decade since we probably could not reclaim more than 15 million acres by drainage and extension of irrigation. The only possibility is to increase the productivity per acre."

I might add that in one of its publications, about two years ago, the United States Department of Agriculture indicated that if our agricultural productivity were at the 1956 level-in other words, if we did adopt some of the measures which would reduce our agricultural productivity to the 1956 levelwe would require some 200 million more acres to feed our 1975 population. How do we increase productivity per acre, and what, if any, is the role of pesticides in bringing about this increase? Well, McNew comments, in part, as follows:

"There are many means of increasing productivity: improved soil fertility, seeding of better varieties, more intensive cultivation, dual cropping, irrigation, etc. However, in any planning for the future the tremendous damage from crop pests looms large. According to the careful survey made by the USDA in 1954, the losses in the United States from insects, diseases, and weeds probably average about 21 per cent of the potential production. This is equivalent to losing 88 million acres of the 358 million acres before they could be harvested. Unfortunately, the losses are not distributed so that they can be disposed of so easily. The inadequate crop has to be harvested, so the farmer loses much of the labor, fertilizer, and equipment expenses he has invested. Any benefits he might have expected from use of extra fertilizers, cultivation or other beneficial practices have automatically been depreciated by the pests. It stands to reason that improvement in the control of pests is the first step toward greater productivity. It is the most direct pathway to realization of all the gains from other production devices.

"There is little need to dwell on the value of pesticides for increasing the yields per acre. The literature is replete with references to the detailed benefits derived from insecticides, fungicides, herbicides and nematocides. The yield increase following application ranges from nothing to complete crop salvage. It is next to impossible to measure these benefits precisely because the results are confounded by many uncontrolled environmental forces, direct effects of the chemical on plants, and even the density of crop stand and supply of available soil nutrients at the time of application. Undoubtedly, the benefits are sometimes overestimated by participating scientists who, in all sincerity and honesty, are impressed by the extreme benefit rather than the average sustained improvement. However, there is plenty of evidence of underestimation of the potential value of pesticides by the biologists who use them, as illustrated by the history of the potato protection in the United States."

Apropos the history of United States potato protection, prior to the 1940's, we were dependent primarily upon Bordeaux mixture fungicide for the control of potato blight. In 1945, the yield was 155 bushels per acre; 2,700,000 acres were harvested. In that year, a pair of new pesticides was introduced. By 1950-in five years-the yield had risen by 100 bushels per acre to 253 bushels per acre, and with a total investment in land of 1,690,000 acresone million less than in 1945-significantly more potatoes were produced. In other words, on something like sixtenths of the land, we were producing more potatoes than we had been, but five years after the introduction of new pesticide control measures.

Comparable statistics have been compiled for many other crops; for example Decker, in "Agricultural Chemicals," in 1954 pointed out that the changes in average yield per acre in the United States in the five years following the introduction of DDT are as follows: field crops which required extensive use of insecticides reflected increased yields of 6.7 to 20 per cent; vegetables exhibited increases from approximately 12 to 62 per cent; and seed yields of legumes rose in the range from 11 to 42 per cent. By contrast, those crops which required scant or no treatment with pesticides during the same period reflected yield increases of, approximately, minus 5 to 6 per cent in field crops, and plus 3 to 6 per cent in vegetables. These correlations are obvious, and, despite the fact that there are many factors involved in recent and ongoing improvements in our scientific agriculture, it is difficult to escape the fact of the tremendous contribution to our food supply of the appropriate and proper use of pesticides.

But what about our present food surpluses? We have all of these surpluseswhy worry about improvements or increases? Well, to cite one year, 1960, the surpluses that at the time appeared to loom so large in political headlines and market economics were in fact no more than approximately 6 per cent of actual usage, and, by 1975, the needs of our population will require 35 to 40 per cent increase in agricultural production over 1960.

What happens to countries-to a country, or to this country-if its agriculture and industry fail to provide an adequate food supply? We do not have to create an imaginary situation to answer this question. We can review our own nutritional history and consider the "good old days" of pellagra, rickets, goiter, protein deficiency, scurvy, higher death rate, shorter life expectancy, and fewer cancers and heart disease because fewer people lived long enough to get them! We can recall, with nostalgia if we would like to, the days of farm animal cultivation, the use of manures as fertilizers, and the so-called simple, tried and true pest control measures.

These coincide, of course, with the days of the home cooked meal and the good life. Or, if we like, we can turn to countries which are at the same stage of development, or even less developed, than we were during those days of our "good life."

I have had the good fortune to have experience in assessing the nutritional problems of a good many countries which are today less fortunate than we are in so far as food supply and nutritional standards are concerned. Let us turn back for a moment to pellagra, a disease which manifests itself in part as a dermatitis of the exposed parts and is caused from a combined deficiency of nicotinic acid and of tryptophane in the diet. This condition frequently arises where diets are primarily composed of maize and corn. In fact, when 60 per cent or more of the calories of a country's or region's diet comes from maize, one can expect to find pellagra. Now, we did have pellagra in this country-the last case of it that I saw in the United States was in Nashville, Tenn., about 12 or 14 years ago.

In Egyptian villages of the Nile Delta, where the diet consists primarily of corn and very little animal protein is consumed, chronic pellagra, with its disfiguring skin lesions and depigmentation, is readily observed. Corn is one of the most readily available sources of food energy, but it has a relatively poor protein content; it constitutes the major item of diet because it is grown more cheaply than other crops due in part to the failure to apply modern scientific agricultural technics.

Similarly, in Yugoslavia, at the height of the pellagra season, 30 per cent of the population manifest lesions of this character. Riboflavin deficiencies occur in many of the same regions-often we see the two conditions in conjunction with one another.

Beriberi, associated with the eating of a different grain, but with the same monotony of diet that causes pellagra, is also a reflection of unsophisticated agricultural development, due to the inability or failure to apply modem agricultural technics which will supply a country with diversified crops and a wide and nutritionally adequate diet selection.

Endemic goiter, we know, is widely prevalent throughout the world. It has largely, though not completely, disappeared in this country, thanks in part to the iodization of salt. This is not the only reason, however, because we have had a complete revolution in the source of our foods, and no longer are those of us who live in iodine-deficient areas dependent for food solely upon the products of our immediate locales. Our food is grown under our concentrated agricultural system, in Florida, South Carolina, New Mexico, Arizona, and elsewhere, and shipped to us. Thus, we have a general mixing of the food supply, and, hence, a leveling out of the amount of iodine in the diet.

In other parts of the world, goiter is so widespread that it is regarded as "normal"- the dolls, even, have goiter in some countries! Other deficiency diseases, such as kwashiorkor, a form of protein malnutrition that is widespread in Asia, Africa, and South America, do not occur in the United States. Xerophthalmia, a form of vitamin A deficiency that is widespread elsewhere, in Indonesia for example, also is unknown here. Yet, in Indonesia a single hospital, which I have visited, has recorded about 1,000 cases annually of this vitamin A deficiency blindness each year for the past decade.

One could go on and on with these deficiency syndromes; iron-deficiency anemia, for example, occurs not only from dietary lack, but at times can almost be called an occupational disease of agricultural workers, because of the exposure to parasitism which is encountered by the agricultural worker in countries infested with bilharziasis. Some of these exposures can be reduced, and are reduced, by proper use of agricultural chemicals.

Growth failure, too, is common among children suffering protein and calorie malnutrition. I have not touched on all of the diseases that are characteristic of these agricultural systems which fail to meet the needs of the people. I could go on for some time just listing them. Rather, I would like to suggest that the responsible scientist, who is concerned with nutrition and health, and with food production and utilization, has an obligation to assure the production and availability of food for the 200 or 220 million people who will be in the United States in 1975, and also for the 3 to 6 per cent increments which are occurring annually in the population in other areas of the world.

As long as society permits an increase in its numbers, it must accept the responsibility for planning, so as to provide adequately for its food supply. In this there is no place for the often made distinction between agriculturally produced and industrially produced foods.

Nor is there a place for those whose nostalgic associations lead them to fear, and thereby to oppose, progress. The scientist's concern is to assure that the rapidly evolving changes of which he is an agent are beneficial, and nonharmful; that the benefits are associated with minimum hazard; and that those who bring forth new developments are aware of their responsibility for proper appraisal of them prior to their widespread application. A major responsibility, therefore, of the scientist concerned with food and nutrition is to assure the fullest, sound application of scientific knowledge, in order to ensure continued availability of adequate, healthful foods.

Bias, bigotry, and faddism must not be permitted to influence laws and regulations in this country in such manner as to interfere with the full use of our nutritional resources, be these resources agricultural or industrial. Neither the interests of irresponsible groups, nor acquiescent reactions to them of responsible ones can be allowed to compromise the nutritional quality of our food supply. Only through widest public understanding of the forces concerned with the provision of our foods, and with the contribution to our abundant, healthful, food supply that is yielded by the many and varied segments of America's resources can we anticipate development that will be the most advantageous to the American public.

10

Chemical and Crop Nutrient Interactions

Micronutrients are regulators, inhibitors and activators of physiological processes, and plants provide a primary dietary source of these elements for animals and people. Micronutrient deficiency symptoms are often indistinct and commonly ascribed to other causes such as drought, extreme temperatures, soil pH, etc. The sporadic nature of distinct visual symptoms, except under severe deficiency conditions, has resulted in a reluctance of many producers to remediate micronutrient deficiency. Lost yield, reduced quality, and increased disease are the unfortunate consequences of untreated micronutrient deficiency. The shift to less tillage, herbicide resistant crops and extensive application of glyphosate has significantly changed nutrient availability and plant efficiency for a number of essential plant nutrients. Some of these changes are through direct toxicity of glyphosate while others are more indirect through changes in soil organisms important for nutrient access, availability, or plant uptake. Compensation for these effects on nutrition can maintain optimum crop production efficiency, maximize yield, improve disease resistance, increase nutritional value, and insure food and feed safety.

Introduction

Thirty+ years ago, U.S. agriculture started a conversion to a monochemical herbicide program focused around glyphosate. The near simultaneous shift from conventional tillage to no-till or minimum tillage stimulated this conversion and the introduction of genetically modified crops tolerant to glyphosate. The introduction of genetically modified Roundup Ready crops has greatly increased the volume and scope of glyphosate usage, and conversion of major segments of crop production to a monochemical herbicide strategy. Interactions of glyphosate with plant nutrition and increased disease have been previously over looked, but become more obvious each year as glyphosate residual effects become more apparent

The extensive use of glyphosate, and the rapid adoption of genetically modified glyphosate-tolerant crops such as soybean, corn, cotton, canola, sugar beets, and alfalfa; with their greatly increased application of glyphosate for simplified weed control, have intensified deficiencies of numerous essential micronutrients and some macronutrients. Additive nutrient inefficiency of the Roundup Ready® (RR) gene and glyphosate herbicide increase the need for micronutrient remediation, and established soil and tissue levels for nutrients considered sufficient for specific crop production may be inadequate indicators in a less nutrient efficient glyphosate weed management program. Understanding glyphosate.s mode of action and impact of the RR gene, indicate strategies to offset negative impacts of this monochemical system on plant nutrition and its predisposition to disease. A basic consideration in this regard should be a much more judicious use of glyphosate. This paper is an update of information on nutrient and disease interactions affected by glyphosate and the RR genes and includes recently published research in the European Journal of Agronomy and other international scientific publications.

Understanding Glyphosate

Glyphosate (N-phosphomonomethyl glycine) is a strong

metal chelator and was first patented as such by Stauffer Chemical Co. in 1964. Metal chelators are used extensively in agriculture to increase solubility or uptake of essential micronutrients that are essential for plant physiological processes. They are also used as herbicides and other biocides nitrification inhibitors, fungicides, plant growth regulators, etc. where they immobilize specific metal co-factors essential for enzyme activity. In contrast to some compounds that chelate with a single or few metal species, glyphosate is a broadspectrum chelator with both macro and micronutrients (Ca, Mg, Cu, Fe, Mn, Ni, Zn). It is this strong, broadspectrum chelating ability that also makes glyphosate a broad-spectrum herbicide and a potent antimicrobial agent since the function of numerous essential enzymes is affected.

Primary emphasis in understanding glyphosate.s herbicidal activity has been on inhibition of the enzyme 5-enolpyruvylshikimate-3-phosphate synthase at the start of the Shikimate physiological pathway for secondary metabolism. This enzyme requires reduced FMN as a co-factor (catalyst) whose reduction requires manganese. Thus, by immobilizing Mn by chelation, glyphosate denies the availability of reduced FMN for the EPSPS enzyme. It also can affect up to 25 other plant enzymes that require Mn as a co-factor and numerous other enzymes in both primary and secondary metabolism that require other metal co-factors. Several of these enzymes also function with Mn in the Shikimate pathway that is responsible for plant responses to stress and defense against pathogens amino acids, hormones, lignin, phytoalexins, flavenoids, phenols, etc. . By inhibiting enzymes in the Shikimate pathway, a plant becomes highly susceptible to various ubiquitous soilborne pathogens (*Fusarium, Pythium, Phytophthora, Rhizoctonia*, etc.). It is this pathogenic activity that actually kills the plant as "the herbicidal mode of action". If glyphosate is not translocated to the roots because of stem boring insects or other disruption of the vascular system, aerial parts of the plant may be stunted, but the plant is not killed.

Recognizing that glyphosate is a strong chelator to

immobilize essential plant micronutrients provides an understanding for the various non-herbicidal and herbicidal effects of glyphosate. Glyphosate is a phloem-mobile, systemic chemical in plants that accumulates in meristematic tissues root, shoot tip, reproductive, legume nodules and is released into the rhizosphere through root exudation from RR as well as non-RR plants or mineralization of treated plant residues. Degradation of glyphosate in most soils is slow or non-existent since it is not „biodegradable. and is primarily by microbial co-metabolism when it does occur. Although glyphosate can be rapidly immobilized in soil also spray tank mixtures, and plants through chelation with various cat-ions it is not readily degraded and can accumulate for years in both soils and perennial plants. Very limited degradation may be a "safety" feature with glyphosate since most degradation products are toxic to normal as well as RR plants. Phosphorus fertilizers can desorb accumulated glyphosate that is immobilized in soil to damage and reduce the physiological efficiency of subsequent crops.

Understanding the Roundup Ready Gene

Plants genetically engineered for glyphosate-tolerance contain the Roundup Ready genes that provide an alternate EPSPS pathway that is not blocked by glyphosate. The purpose of these gene inserts is to provide herbicidal selectivity so glyphosate can be applied directly to these plants rather than only for preplant applications. As an additional physiological mechanism, activity of this duplicate pathway requires energy from the plant that could be used for yield. The RR genes are „silent. in meristematic tissues where glyphosate accumulates so that these rapidly metabolizing tissues are not provided an active alternative EPSPS pathway to counter the physiological effects of glyphosate.s inhibition of EPSPS. Meristematic tissues also are areas of high physiologic activity requiring a higher availability of the essential micronutrients needed for cell division and growth that glyphosate immobilizes by chelation.

Residual glyphosate in RR plant tissues can immobilize Fe, Mn, Zn or other nutrients applied as foliar amendments for 8-

35 days after it has been applied. This reduces the availability of micronutrients required for photosynthesis, disease resistance, and other critical physiological functions.The presence of the RR gene(s) reduces nutrient uptake and physiological efficiency and may account for some of the „yield drag. reported for RR crops when compared with the „normal. isolines from which they were derived. Reduced physiological efficiency from the RR gene is also reflected in reduced water use efficiency and increased drought stress.

It should be recognized that there is nothing in the glyphosate-tolerant plant that operates on the glyphosate applied to the plant. All the technology does is insert an alternative enzyme (EPSPS-II) that is not blocked by glyphosate in mature tissue. Thus, when glyphosate enters the plant, it is not selective; it chelates with a host of elements influencing nutrient availability, disease resistance, and the plant's other physiological functions for the life of the plant or until it is exuded into soil or groundwater through the roots.

Interactions of Glyphosate with Plant Nutrition

Glyphosate can affect nutrient efficiency in the plant by chelating essential nutrient co-factors after application since there is 100 to 1000 times more „free. glyphosate in the plant than all of the unbound cat-ions. Chelation of Mn and other micronutrients after application of glyphosate is frequently observed as a „flashing. or yellowing that persists until the plant can resupply. the immobilized nutrients. The duration of flashing. is correlated with the availability of micronutrients in soil. Symptom remission indicates a resumption of physiological processes, but is not an indicator of plant nutrient sufficiency since micronutrient deficiencies are commonly referred to as „hidden hunger.. As a strong nutrient chelator, glyphosate can reduce physiological efficiency by immobilizing elements required as components, co-factors or regulators of physiological functions at very low rates. Thus, plant uptake and or translocation of Fe, Mn and Zn are drastically reduced by commonly observed „drift. rates of glyphosate. This is reflected in reduced physiological efficiency, lower mineral nutrient levels in vegetative and reproductive tissues, and increased susceptibility to disease. Microbial and plant production of siderophores and ferric reductase in root exudates under nutrient stress are inhibited by glyphosate to exacerbate plant nutrient stress common in low-available micronutrient soils.

Glyphosate is not readily degraded in soil and can probably accumulate for many years chelated with soil cat-ions. Degradation products of glyphosate are as damaging to RR crops as to non-RR crops. Persistence and accumulation of glyphosate in perennial plants, soil, and root meristems, can significantly reduce root growth and the development of nutrient absorptive tissue of RR as well as non-RR plants to further impair nutrient uptake and efficiency. Impaired root uptake not only reduces the availability of specific nutrients, but also affects the natural ability of plants to compensate for low levels of many other nutrients. Glyphosate also reduces nutrient uptake from soil indirectly through its toxicity to many soil microorganisms responsible for increasing the availability and access to nutrients through mineralization, reduction, symbiosis, etc.

Degradation of plant tissues through growth, necrosis, or mineralization of residues can release accumulated glyphosate from meristematic tissues in toxic concentrations to plants. The most damaging time to plant wheat in ryegrass „burned down. by glyphosate is two weeks after glyphosate application to correspond with the release of accumulated glyphosate from decomposing meristematic tissues. This is contrasted with the need to delay seeding of winter wheat for 2-3 weeks after a regular weed burn-down. to permit time for immobilization of glyphosate from root exudates and direct application through chelation with soil cat-ions. The Roundup® label for Israel lists recommended waiting times before planting a susceptible crop on that soil.

One of the benefits of crop rotation is an increased availability of nutrients for a subsequent crop in the rotation. The high level of available Mn (130 ppm) after a normal corn crop is not observed after glyphosate-treated RR corn. The lower nutrient availability after specific RR crop sequences may need to be compensated for through micronutrient application in order to optimize yield and reduce disease in a subsequent crop.

The Influence of Glyphosate on Soil Organisms Important for Access Mineralization, Solubilization and Fixation of Essential Plant Nutrients

Glyphosate is a potent microbiocide and is toxic to earthworms, mycorrhizae, reducing microbes that convert insoluble soil oxides to plant available forms (Mn and Fe, *Pseudomonads, Bacillus*, etc.), nitrogen-fixing organisms (*Bradyrhizobium, Rhizobium*), and organisms involved in the „natural,. biological control of soilborne diseases that reduce root uptake of nutrients. Although glyphosate contact with these organisms is limited by rapid chelation-immobilization when applied on fallow soil; glyphosate in root exudates, or from decaying weed tissues or RR plants, contacts these organisms in their most active ecological habitat throughout the rhizosphere. It is not uncommon to see Cu, Fe, Mg, Mn, Ni, and Zn deficiencies intensify and show in soils that were once considered fully sufficient for these nutrients. Increasing the supply and availability of Co, Cu, Fe, Mg, Mn, Ni, and Zn have reduced some of the deleterious effects of glyphosate on these organisms and increased crop yields.

In contrast to microbial toxicity, glyphosate in soil and root exudates stimulates oxidative soil microbes that reduce nutrient availability by decreasing their solubility for plant uptake, immobilize nutrients such as K in microbial sinks to deny availability for plants, and deny access to soil nutrients through pathogenic activity. Plant pathogens stimulated by glyphosate include ubiquitous bacterial and fungal root, crown, and stalk rotting fungi; vascular colonizing organisms that disrupt nutrient transport to cause wilt and die-back; and root nibblers that impair access or uptake of soil nutrients.

Herbicidal Mode of Action of Glyphosate

As a strong metal micronutrient chelator, glyphosate inhibits activity of EPSPS and other enzymes in the Shikimate metabolic pathway responsible for plant resistance to various pathogens. Plant death is through greatly increased plant susceptibility of non-RR plants to common soilborne fungi such as *Fusarium, Rhizoctonia, Pythium, Phytophthora,* etc. that are also stimulated by glyphosate. It is very difficult to kill a plant in sterile soil by merely shutting down the Shikimate pathway secondary metabolism unless soilborne pathogens are also present. It is the increased susceptibility to soilborne pathogens, and increased virulence of the pathogens, that actually kills the plants after applying glyphosate. Disease resistance in plants is manifest through various active and passive physiological mechanisms requiring micronutrients. Those metabolic pathways producing secondary anti-microbial compounds phytoalexins, flavenoids, etc., pathogen inhibiting amino acids and peptides, hormones involved in cicatrisation walling off pathogens, callusing, and disease escape mechanisms can all be compromised by glyphosate chelation of micronutrient co-factors critical for enzyme function. Genetic modification of plants for glyphosate tolerance partially restores Shikimate pathway function to provide a selective herbicidal effect.

Interactions of Glyphosate with Plant Disease

Micronutrients are the regulators, activators, and inhibitors of plant defense mechanisms that provide resistance to stress and disease. Chelation of these nutrients by glyphosate compromises plant defenses and increases pathogenesis to increase the severity of many abiotic (bark cracking, nutrient deficiencies) as well as infectious diseases of both RR and non-plants in the crop production system (table 4). Many of these diseases are referred to as „emerging. or reemerging. diseases because they rarely caused economic losses in the past, or were effectively controlled through management practices.

Non-infectious (Abiotic) Diseases: Research at Ohio State

University has shown that bark cracking, sunscald, and winter-kill of trees and perennial ornamentals is caused by glyphosate used for under-story weed control, and that glyphosate can accumulate for 8-10 years in perennial plants. This accumulation of glyphosate can be from the inadvertent uptake of glyphosate from contact with bark or by root uptake from glyphosate in weed root exudates in soil. Severe glyphosate damage to trees adjacent to stumps of cut trees treated with glyphosate to prevent sprouting in an effort to eradicate citrus greening or CVC can occur through root translocation and exudation several years after tree removal.

Infectious Diseases: Increased severity of the take-all root and crown rot of cereals (*Gaeumannomyces graminis*) after prior glyphosate usage has been observed for over 20 years and take-all is now a „reemerging. disease in many wheat producing areas of the world where glyphosate is used for weed control prior to cereal planting. A related disease of cereals, and the cause of rice blast (*Magnaporthe grisea*), is becoming very severe in Brazil and is especially severe when wheat follows a RR crop in the rotation. Like take-all and Fusarium root rot, this soilborne pathogen also infects wheat and barley roots, and is a concern for U.S. cereal production.

Fusarium species causing head scab are common root and crown rot pathogens of cereals everywhere; however, Fusarium head scab has generally been a serious disease of wheat and barley only in warm temperate regions of the U.S. With the extensive use of glyphosate, it is now of epidemic proportions and prevalent throughout most of the cereal producing areas of North America. Canadian research has shown that the application of glyphosate one or more times *in the three years previous to planting wheat* was the most important agronomic factor associated with high FHB in wheat, with a 75 % increase in FHB for all crops and a 122 % increase for crops under minimum-till where more glyphosate is used. The most severe FHB occurs where a RR crop precedes wheat in the rotation for the same reason. Glyphosate altered plant physiology (carbon and nitrogen metabolism) increasing susceptibility of wheat and barley to FHB and increased toxin production, is also associated with a transient tolerance of wheat and soybeans to rust diseases.

The increased FHB with glyphosate results in a dramatic increase in tricothecene (deoxynivalenol, nivalenol, „vomitoxins.) and estrogenic (zaeralenone) mycotoxins in grain; however, the high concentrations of mycotoxin in grain are not always associated with *Fusarium* infection of kernels. Quite often overlooked is the increase in root and crown rot by FHB *Fusaria* with glyphosate and the production of mycotoxins in root and crown tissues with subsequent translocation to stems, chaff and grain. Caution has been expressed in using straw and chaff as bedding for pigs or roughage for cattle because of mycotoxin levels that far exceeded clinically significant levels for infertility and toxicity. This also poses a health and safety concern for grain entering the food chain for humans. The list of diseases affected by glyphosate (see reference No. 18) is increasing as growers and pathologists recognize the cause-effect relationship.

Special Nutrient Considerations in a Glyphosate Dominant Weed Management Ecological System

There are two things that should be understood in order to remediate nutrient deficiencies in a glyphosate usage program: 1) the effects of glyphosate on nutrient availability and function and 2) the effect of the RR gene on nutrient efficiency. With this understanding, there are four objectives for fertilization in a glyphosate environment all of which indicate a more judicious use of glyphosate as part of the remediation process. These four objectives are to:

1. Provide adequate nutrient availability for full functional sufficiency to compensate for glyphosate and RR reduced availability or physiological efficiency of micronutrients.

2. Detoxify residual glyphosate in meristematic and other tissues, in root exudates, and in soil by adding

appropriate elements for chelation with the residual glyphosate.

3. Restore soil microbial activity to enhance nutrient availability, supply, and balance that are inhibited by residual glyphosate in soil and glyphosate in root exudates.

4. Increase plant resistance to root infecting and reemerging diseases through physiological plant defense mechanisms dependent on the Shikimate, amino acid, and other pathways that are compromised by micronutrient inefficiency in a glyphosate environment.

Meeting Nutrient Sufficiency: Extensive research has shown that increased levels and availability of micronutrients such as Mn, Zn, Cu, Fe, Ni, etc can compensate for reduced nutrient efficiency and the inefficiency of RR crops. This need may not be manifest in high fertility or nutrient toxic soils for a few years after moving to a predominantly monochemical strategy. The timing for correcting micronutrient deficiencies is generally more critical for cereal plants (barley, corn, wheat) than for legumes in order to prevent irreversible yield and or quality loss. Nutrient sufficiency levels from soil and tissue analysis that are considered adequate for non-GM crops may need to be increased for RR crops to be at full physiological sufficiency. Since residual „free. glyphosate in RR plant tissues can immobilize most regular sources of foliar-applied micronutrients for 8-15 days, and thereby reduce the future availability of these materials, it may be best to apply some micronutrients 1-2 weeks after glyphosate is applied to RR crops.

The expense of an additional trip across the field for foliar application frequently deters micronutrient fertilization for optimum crop yield and quality. There are newly available micronutrient formulations (nutrient phosphites) that maintain plant availability without impacting herbicidal activity of the glyphosate in a tank-mix, and plants have responded well from these micronutrient-glyphosate mixes. Simultaneous application of some micronutrients with glyphosate might provide an efficient means to overcome deficiencies in low fertility soils, as well as mitigate the reduced physiological efficiency inherent with the glyphosate-tolerant gene and glyphosate immobilization of essential nutrients in the plant.

Under severe micronutrient deficiency conditions, selecting seed high in nutrient content or a micronutrient seed treatment to provide early nutrient sufficiency, establish a well-developed root system, and insure a vigorous seedling plant with increased tolerance to glyphosate applied later, has been beneficial even though excess nutrient applied at this time may be immobilized by glyphosate from root exudates and not available for subsequent plant uptake. Micronutrients such as Mn are not efficiently broadcast applied to soil for plant uptake because of microbial immobilization to non-available oxidized Mn, but could be applied in a band or to seed or foliage.

Detoxifying Residual Glyphosate: Some nutrients are relatively immobile in plant tissues so that a combination of micronutrients may be more beneficial than any individual one to chelate with residual glyphosate and „detoxify. it in meristematic and mature tissues. Thus, foliar application of Mn could remediate for glyphosate immobilization of the nutrient; however, it may be more effective when applied in combination with the more mobile Zn to detoxify sequestered glyphosate in meristematic tissues even though Zn levels may appear sufficient. Gypsum applied in the seed row has shown some promise for detoxifying glyphosate from root exudates since Ca is a good chelator with glyphosate (one of the reasons that ammonium sulfate is recommended in spray solutions with hard water is to prevent chelation with Ca and Mg which would inhibit herbicidal activity.

Although bioremediation of accumulating glyphosate in soil may be possible in the future, initial degradation products of glyphosate are toxic to both RR and non-RR plants. This is an area that needs greater effort since the application of phosphorus fertilizers can desorb immobilized glyphosate to be toxic to plants through root uptake. Micronutrient seed treatment can provide some detoxification during seed germination, and stimulate vigor and root growth to enhance recovery from later glyphosate applications.

Biological Remediation: The selection and use of plants for glyphosate-tolerance that have greater nutrient efficiency for uptake or physiological function has improved the performance of some RR crops, and further improvements are possible in this area. Enhancing soil microbial activity to increase nutrient availability and plant uptake has been possible through seed inoculation, environmental modification to favor certain groups of organisms, and implementation of various management practices. There are many organisms that have been used to promote plant growth, with the most recognized being legume inoculants (*Rhizobia, Bradyrhizobia* species); however, glyphosate is toxic to these beneficial microorganisms. Continued use of glyphosate in a cereal-legume rotation has greatly reduced the population of these organisms in soil so that annual inoculation of legume seed is frequently recommended.

Biological remediation to compensate for glyphosate.s impact on soil organisms important in nutrient cycles may be possible if the remediating organism is also glyphosate-tolerant and capable of over coming the soils natural biological buffering capacity. This would be especially important for nitrogen-fixing, mycorrhizae, and mineral reducing organisms, but will be of limited benefit unless the introduced organisms are also tolerant of glyphosate. Modification of the soil biological environment through tillage, crop sequence, or other cultural management practices might also be a viable way to stimulate the desired soil biological activity.

Increasing Plant Resistance to Stress and Root-Infecting Pathogens: Maintaining plant health is a basic requirement for crop yield and quality. Plant tolerance to stress and many pathogens is dependent on a full sufficiency of micronutrients to maintain physiological processes mediated through the Shikimate or other pathways that are compromised in a glyphosate environment. Sequential application(s) of specific micronutrients (esp. Ca, Cu, Fe, Mn, Zn) may be required to compensate for those nutrients physiologically lost through glyphosate chelation. Breeding for increased nutrient efficiency and disease resistance will be an important contributor to this objective.

Glyphosate is a strong, broad-spectrum nutrient chelator that inhibits plant enzymes responsible for disease resistance so that plants succumb from pathogenic attack. This also predisposes RR and non-RR plants to other pathogens. The introduction of such an intense mineral chelator as glyphosate into the food chain through accumulation in feed, forage, and food, and root exudation into ground water, could pose significant health concerns for animals and humans and needs further evaluation. Chelation immobilization of such essential elements as Ca, Fe (blood), Mn, Zn (liver, kidney), Cu, Mg (brain) could directly inhibit vital functions and predispose to disease. The lower mineral nutrient content of feeds and forage from a glyphosate-intense weed management program can generally be compensated for through mineral supplementation.

11

Earthworms Vermicompost: A Powerful Crop Nutrient

Introduction

Earthworms vermicompost is proving to be highly nutritive 'organic fertilizer' and more powerful 'growth promoter' over the conventional composts and a 'protective' farm input (increasing the physical, chemical & biological properties of soil, restoring & improving its natural fertility) against the 'destructive' chemical fertilizers which has destroyed the soil properties and decreased its natural fertility over the years. Vermicompost is rich in NKP nitrogen 2-3%, potassium 1.85-2.25% and phosphorus 1.55-2.25%, micronutrients, beneficial soil microbes and also contain 'plant growth hormones & enzymes'. It is scientifically proving as 'miracle growth promoter & also plant protector' from pests and diseases. Vermicompost retains nutrients for long time and while the conventional compost fails to deliver the required amount of macro and micronutrients including the vital NKP to plants in shorter time, the vermicompost does.

Protective Compost Versus the Destructive Chemical Fertilizers

Chemical fertilizers which ushered the 'green revolution' in the 1950-60's came as a 'mixed blessing' for mankind. It boosted food productivity, but at the cost of environment & society. It dramatically increased the 'quantity' of the food produced but decreased its 'nutritional quality' and also the 'soil fertility' over the years. It killed the beneficial soil organisms which help in renewing natural fertility. It also impaired the power of 'biological resistance' in crops making them more susceptible to pests & diseases. Over the years it has worked like a 'slow poison' for the soil with a serious 'withdrawal symptoms'. The excessive use of 'nitrogenous fertilizer' (urea) has also led to increase in the level of 'inorganic nitrogen' content in groundwater (through leaching effects) and in the human food with grave consequences for the human health. Chemically grown foods have adversely affected human health.

Organic farming systems with the aid of various nutrients of biological origin such as compost are thought to be the answer for the 'food safety and farm security' in future. Among them 'composts' made from biodegradation of organics of MSW which is being generated in huge amount every day all over the world are most important. The organic fraction of the MSW (about 70-80%) containing plenty of nitrogen (N), potash (K) and phosphorus (P) is a good source of macro and micronutrients for the soil. Composts also contain plenty of 'beneficial soil microbes' which help in 'soil regeneration' & 'fertility improvement' and protect them from degradation while also promoting growth in plants Composts also protect plants from pests and diseases.

Properties of farm soil using compost vis-a-vis chemical fertilizers: Suhane studied the chemical and biological properties of soil under organic farming using various types of composts and chemical farming using chemical fertilizers-urea (N), phosphates (P) and potash (K). All compost including vermicompost, are produced from some 'waste materials' of society which is converted into a 'valuable resource'. It is like 'killing two birds in one shot'. More significant is that it is of biological origin i.e. a 'renewable resource' and will be readily available to mankind in future. Whereas, chemical fertilizers are made from petroleum products which are 'non-renewable' and a 'depleting' resource.

Integrated Plant Nutrient Management in crop production in the Central Ethiopian highlands.

Ethiopia is located in east Africa between 3 N and 15 N latitudes and 33 E and 48 E longitudes. The country covers an altitude range from 126 meters below sea level to 4620 m.a.s.l.. Ethiopia has an area of 1.13 million km^2 and occupies a huge landmass of Africa. Characteristically it has a rugged landscape, from a highland complex of mountains and bisected plateaux at the heart to torrid plains. Though the country is found in the tropics, the highlands enjoy temperate and tropical climates. The altitude modifies the temperatures and the annual average is seldom higher than 20C. Most of the highlands have rainfall in the range of 600 to 2700 mm.

The Ethiopian highlands are one of the hotspots on the African continent with regard to food production and in the struggle to preserve the natural resource base. The Ethiopian highlands cover 95% of the cropped area in Ethiopia and contain almost 85% of the Ethiopian population.

The cropped area is subject to severe losses of nutrients through soil erosion and by removal of dung and crop residue for fuel. Nutrient balance calculations for countries by Stoorvogel and Smaling showed that Ethiopia was among the countries with the highest rates of net nutrient losses. The annual nutrient deficit is estimated at -41 kg N, -6 kg P and -26 kg K ha`

In the Ethiopian highland soil loss due to water erosion is about 1493 million ton per annum as estimated by Hurni (1993). Of this, nearly half is estimated to come from cultivated fields, which account for only about 13% of the country's total area. These losses will inevitably cause yield decreases unless appropriate measures are taken.

Population growth rate is high and by the year 2020 is expected to exceed 110 million, which is about a doubling of the current population. If present production trends remain unchanged, Ethiopia will face a food deficit. However, this negative trend can be reverted if appropriate measures are taken. Most Ethiopian soils are deficit in nutrients, especially nitrogen and phosphorus and fertilizer application has significantly increased yields of crops.

However, despite the potential for increasing yields and farm income by the use of fertilizer, many small scale and poor farmers do not have the resources to make use of fertilizer for various reasons.

Hence, it is important to understand these constraints and develop low cost technologies that focus on development of appropriate Integrated Plant Nutrient Management for the Ethiopian highlands. Integrated Plant Nutrient Management is based on the principles i) optimising the use of organic fertiliser ii) supplementing with mineral fertiliser when needed and iii) minimising losses of nutrients. IPNM is not only concerned with good agronomy, but its success is highly dependent on economic, social and institutional issues.

The objectives

The overall objective of this research was to understand the dynamics of soil nutrients and their management at farm level and to develop participatory plant nutrient management options for sustainable production.

Approach

The study employed different approaches: household survey with formal questionnaire, focus group discussion, interviews, household nutrient flow monitoring, participatory on farm experiments, on farm experiment, on-station field and greenhouse experiments.

Participatory nutrient flow monitoring

Quantitative analysis of nutrient-flow processes at farms of different socio economic levels was carried out to identify hotspots of soil nutrient depletion and suggest options for soil nutrient maintenance in Gare Arera farming systems.

Participatory on-farm experiments

Three participatory on-farm experiments were carried out. The first experiment was carried out to identify, characterize and evaluate the organic nutrient sources available in Gare Arera. The second experiment evaluated the performance of conservation tillage in tef and wheat in Vertisol and Nitosol in Gare arera.

The third experiment was carried out to monitor the N use efficiency of urea fertilizer applied to tef under farmers' management in East Shawa zone.

On-station experiment

A field experiment was carried out to evaluate mustard meal as a source of N on tef at Holetta.

Greenhouse experiments

A series of greenhouse experiments was carried out to study the effect of key factors on fertilizer N use efficiency of tef.

Nutrient balance at farm, soil fertility class and crop levels

The result of the nutrient flow and balance study showed significant difference in nutrient inputs outputs and balances between farms and within a farm. One important finding was that it matters at which scale nutrient balance is studied. The nutrient balance at the farm level was more positive than at the plot and crop levels. The reason was that nutrients accumulated in deposition sites in the vicinity of the homestead.

The highest depletion was on very poor fertility soils as the land use of these soils was either a crop with low value or grazing land. Good and medium fertility soils are planted mostly with high value crops. Nevertheless the nutrient balance on all the crops, including tef was negative due to low nutrient input, high biomass removal and N losses. In all farms the most severe nutrient depletion was on grasslands.

There are options for increasing nutrient input from cheap nutrient sources such as farmyard and manure, compost, N fixation and bone meal application. Minimum tillage, safe removal of excess water from cropland and gully stabilization can reduce nutrient loses.

Comparative effect of urea and organic nutrient sources on tef

Major organic nutrient sources available at household level in the area were identified, characterised and evaluated. Application of organic material N at equivalent rate to tef on Nitosol and Vertisols resulted in the mean grain yield of 82 % and 99 % of urea treatment yield respectively. The apparent N recovery of urea and the organic materials was 27 and 21 respectively. The agronomic efficiency of the organic fertilizers was similar to urea on the Vertisol. The agro-ecological conditions in the study area appear favourable for the use of organic materials. ANR of urea was low, the surface broadcasting of urea and the high rainfall at time of application might have favoured N losses through different pathways. On Vertisol, tef was more responsive to FYM and on the Nitosol to compost. Compost enriched with ash could be a good choice on Nitosol while FYM performed well on Vertisol. Mustard meal can be applied on both soils in the vicinity of its production. The calculated average annual manure production per household varied from 2866 kg for poor farmers to 11653 kg for rich farmers. N calculated based on mustard seed production in Ethiopia in 2000 was about 580 Mg or 2.8 % of the total urea N consumption in Ethiopia (FAO 2004) during the same period.

Mustard meal N uptake by tef evaluated (paper 3)

When N uptake from mustard meal and urea mixed in different ratios was studied with N technique, the mean N use efficiency from urea was 40 % and was not affected by ratio of mustard meal. The mean % N use efficiency from mustard meal was 22.

NUE of tef monitored

When the fertiliser N use efficiency from urea applied to tef on Vertisol and Andosol was monitored under farmers' field management condition, the FNUE on Andosol was 33% compared to 22% on Vertisols. Higher uptake on Andosol was may be due to better soil drainage.

Urea and ammonium sulphate N use efficiency of four tef varieties studied under greenhouse conditions on typic Eutrocrept soil showed higher % FNUE for all the tested tef varieties when the N source was urea compared to ammonium sulphate. The mean % FNUE for urea and ammonium sulphate was 48 and 34% respectively. When the varieties were grown on a Nitosol or a Vertisol and ammonium sulphate was applied, the % FNUE of the tef varieties was 61% on the Nitosol and 28% on the Vertisol.

Option of zero and reduced tillage in tef and wheat production

The study assessed agronomic and economic effect of conventional tillage four times ploughing, reduced tillage one time pass with the plough, zero tillage and Broad Bed Furrow. Farmers' perceptions on the methods were in addition assessed. The results showed that one time ploughing could be an option to conventional ploughing in tef, as there was no significant difference in yields and gross margin on the Vertisol. On the Nitosol, though there was no difference in the yield, the gross margin on minimum tillage was lower than the conventional. Nevertheless, the benefit of minimum tillage is not only the immediate economical benefit. BBF gave the highest yield of wheat on Vertisols followed by minimum tillage.

The willingness of farmers to adopt the zero reduced tillage was low but varied with age and sex. Minimum tillage is an interesting option particularly for female headed households because it will reduce the need to rent oxen. Reduced tillage zero tillage will also improve overall productivity of the farming system because it allows partly replacing oxen with cows and reduces the soil erosion.

Contribution of the study to Integrated Plant Nutrient Management in Ethiopia

IPNM seeks both increased agricultural production and preservation of the environment for future generations. IPNM relies on nutrient application and conservation, new technologies to increase nutrient availability to plants, and the dissemination of knowledge between farmers, researchers and other stakeholders.

The nutrient flow analysis study in this work identified the unbalanced nutrient input and output and indicated the soil nutrient reserve was depleting. As reserves get depleted, crop growth and productivity could be compromised. The study showed that there is a scope for better management of organic nutrient sources.

Increased agricultural production through increased nutrient application is among IPNM strategies. In this work the possibility for increased nutrient input from locally available sources to the farming system were assessed in a survey and organic nutrient sources were identified. The identified nutrient sources were evaluated and their effect compared with mineral fertilizer. Composting was introduced as new technology to increase nutrient availability to plants and minimize constraints connected with manure use

Conservation tillage that minimizes soil disturbance and soil erosion was studied and the possibility of sowing tef and wheat with minimum tillage was suggested.

The study showed that that there is no panacea to improved IPNM in the Ethiopian highlands. Choices of IPNM method depend on wealth and gender of farmers, position of the field, crops grown, soil type, access to manure and mineral fertilisers. All these factors vary between the farms.

Rich and medium wealth group farmers could afford to

apply mineral fertilizers and increase nutrient inputs from organic sources as they have more access to manure and other organic materials for compost production. They can apply farmyard manure on Vertisols and ash enriched compost on Nitosol.

Poor farmers do not have many choices in the absence of a credit scheme. They have to increase nutrient input from cheap sources by incorporating more N fixing crops in the crop rotation and producing ash enriched compost.

Female farmers and poor male farmers without oxen have the option to use minimum tillage to reduce the ploughing cost. Similarly reduced tillage can be an alternative on soils prone to soil erosion. Advice to farmer with regard to IPNM must try to reflect this diversity in farmers' wealth and agro-ecological conditions.

This study sought to involve farmers strongly in the research and development process. Farmers were involved in nutrient monitoring, training and in discussion forums between government and non-governmental representatives, researchers and farmers. IPNM requires intensive knowledge dissemination between farmers and other stakeholders.

This study did not address the full range of factors that influence IPNM in the Ethiopian highlands. Further studies are needed to get a more comprehensive picture on the factors that influence agricultural practices and nutrient management in Ethiopia highlands. Nevertheless, I assume that this study should give a contribution to how future IPNM strategies could take into consideration local agronomic, social and economic issues.

12

Integrated Nutrient Management for Sustainable Crop Production

Laboratory, growth chamber and multiyear field studies were conducted with prominent cropping systems of the subtropical northwestern states of India including rice-wheat, rice-mustard, rice-rapeseed, soybean--wheat, soybean rapeseed, groundnut–wheat, and groundnut–sunflower by including legumes moongbean, cowpea, sesbania, pigeon pea to investigate the role of integrated nutrient management in harnessing economically-viable sustainable production, enhancing nutritive quality of the produce, improving soil health, and minimizing environmental pollution. Besides growing legumes and short-duration pulse crops in crop rotations, the effects of integrated use of organics farmyard manure, piggery manure, poultry manure, green manures and crop residues with chemical fertilizers, and impacts of long-term use of INM on enhancing crop productivity were studied. The results clearly demonstrated that INM enhances the yield potential of crops over and above achievable yield with recommended fertilizers, and results in better synchrony of crop N needs due to (a) slower mineralization of organics, (b) reduced N losses via denitrification and nitrate leaching, enhanced nutrient use efficiency and recovery by crops, and improvements in soil health and productivity, and hence could sustain high crop yields in various cropping systems ensuring long-term sustainability of the system.

Introduction

One of the most important challenges facing humanity today is to conserve sustain natural resources, including soil and water, for increasing food production while protecting the environment. As the world population grows, stress on natural resources increases, making it difficult to maintain food security. Longterm food security requires a balance between increasing crop production, maintaining soil health and environmental sustainability. In India, effective nutrient management has played a major role in accomplishing the enormous increase in foodgrain production from 52 million tons in 1951-52 to 230 million tons during 2007-08. However, application of imbalanced and or excessive nutrients led to declining nutrient-use efficiency making fertilizer consumption uneconomical and producing adverse effects on atmosphere and groundwater quality causing health hazards and climate change. On other hand, nutrient mining has occurred in many soils due to lack of affordable fertilizer sources and where fewer or no organic residues are returned to the soils.

Arid and semiarid subtropical soils of northwestern states of India, developed under harsh climate, are inherently poor in organic matter, fertility and water-holding capacity. In these soils, N, P and S deficiencies are principal yield-limiting factors for crop production. INM, which entails the maintenance adjustment of soil fertility to an optimum level for crop productivity to obtain the maximum benefit from all possible sources of plant nutrients - organics as well as inorganics - in an integrated manner, is an essential step to address the twin concerns of nutrient excess and nutrient depletion. INM is also important for marginal farmers who cannot afford to supply crop nutrients through costly chemical fertilizers. This paper summarizes the results of extensive research work carried out with dominant crop rotations of major field crops grown in the subtropical northwestern states of India to investigate the role of INM in harnessing economically-viable sustainable production of prominent cropping systems, enhancing nutritive quality of the produce, improving soil health, and minimizing environmental pollution.

Methods

The subtropical regions of northwestern states of India have summer and winter crop-growing seasons where summer is characterized by high temperature and rainfall the winter is often dry with low temperature, which is suitable for growing field crops under irrigated conditions. The application of organic manures and raising leguminous crops for green manure are generally followed in summer crops, as 2010 19th World Congress of Soil Science, Soil Solutions for a Changing World 80 1 – 6 August 2010, Brisbane, Australia. Published on DVD. the temperature and moisture conditions are favourable. Several laboratory, growth chamber and field studies were conducted to study the effects of growing legumes and short-duration pulse crops in crop rotations, integrated use of organics farmyard manure piggery manure, poultry manure, GM and crop residue with chemical fertilizers, and impacts of long-term use of INM on enhancing crop productivity.

Dominant crop rotations of major field crops such as rice–wheat, rice–mustard, rice–rapeseed, soybean– wheat, soybean–rapeseed, groundnut–wheat, and groundnut–sunflower were studied. Leguminous crops (sesbania, cowpea, mungbean), which accumulate biomass at a rapid rate, were grown when fields were vacant and incorporated into soil at or near flowering as GM. Crop yields and nutrients uptake, transformations and leaching of nutrients in soil, gaseous N losses and denitrification, leaching of nutrients, biological N fixation by legumes estimated using 15N dilution technique, soil quality parameters such as available nutrients, SOC, water soluble C, particulate organic matter C, light fraction organic matter C, microbial biomass C, and conserved soil moisture were measured.

Results

Studies conducted under controlled conditions in growth

chamber and laboratory revealed that (a) mineralization of nutrients from added organics was differentially affected by temperature, soil aeration status, crop residue quality, and soil P status, (b) the nutrient release pattern and mineralization were directly related to N, P and S content of organics and inversely to carbon to nutrient ratios; thereby implying that a crop residue with high nutrient concentration and lower C:Nutrient ratio decomposes easily and releases nutrient at fast rate, (c) high N, P or S concentration in crop residue reduces the competition for soil mineral nutrient by microorganisms and thus enhances the decomposition by supporting higher microbial activity, (d) provided evidence that the C:N, C:P and C:S ratios are reliable and simple to determine for describing crop residue quality, (e) organics enhanced denitrification losses from soils under nearly-saturated and flooded conditions, and (f) CO2 emission from soils, an indicator of C supply to microorganisms, was directly related to denitrification activity. Verification of these findings under field conditions confirmed that (a) sesbania

GM that had high N content and narrow C:N ratio mineralized rapidly, which explained the enhanced efficiency of GM, compared to fertilizer N in supplying N to growing plants and increasing crop yields, N uptake, and N recovery; (b) wide C:N ratio crop residues of wheat, rice and rapeseed caused immobilization of mineral N but with conjoint incorporation of sesbania GM counteracted this deleterious effect, supplied N to rice and increased yields; and (c) incorporation of narrow C:N ratio groundnut residues in conjunction with fertilizer N and P in sunflower crop exhibited fast N and P mineralization even during cool winter; 31 % of groundnut residue-N and 32 % of groundnut residue-P were utilized by the crops, and Olsen-P status of soil increased from initial 12 kg P / ha to 24–43 kg P / ha in INM plots after 4 years of groundnut-sunflower rotation.

However, few revelations noted under controlled conditions, where moisture and temperature regimes were kept constant and plants were not grown, were not observed under field conditions. (a) While organics such as GM, FYM and CR increased N2O emissions under laboratory conditions, INM did not affect N2O emissions in rice-wheat rotation under field conditions. (b) Application of organics in conjunction with FN enhanced denitrification losses from soils under nearly-saturated and flooded conditions under controlled conditions, whereas INM significantly reduced gaseous N losses as compared to the application of FN alone in rice-wheat system. (c) No doubt the increased CO2 production with INM in soils under rice coincided with enhanced rates of denitrification but the total flux of CO2-C from rice-wheat system even with the use of organics was far less than CO2-C consumed by crops for photosynthesis suggesting that high yielding cropping systems are rather sinks than sources of atmospheric CO2-C. This research work further illustrated that (a) INM significantly improves physical, chemical and biological properties of soil; (b) depending upon the ease of mineralization as related to C:N ratio of added organics, 6 % of added C through sesbania GM, 10 % of groundnut residues, 17 % of rice residue and 21 % of wheat residue was sequestered into the soil in a period of 4 years; (c) SOC and other labile pools of C and N were significantly improved with INM plots after 4 years of study (d) while FN had no residual effects, residual GM produced significantly greater yields of a succeeding crop due to the supply of N equivalent to 17-90 kg FN/ha in different crop rotations; for example, GM could save up to 60 kg N/ha in rice and 30 kg N/ha in succeeding wheat or 17 kg N/ha in rapeseed; (e) surface retained crop residues in no-till field conserved soil moisture and enhanced the intrinsic biological N-fixing capacity of soybean by 20 % hus enabling legumes to meet the large proportion of their N requirement; and (f) INM enhanced crop quality by enhancing the acquisition of nutrients, synthesis of protein, oil and fatty acids.

The findings on microbial transformations of organic amendments to plant available N, P and S, and gaseous N forms led to the better understanding of N cycling processes to develop most efficient use of organics for the (a) evaluation of agricultural management effects on soil health and productivity, (b) determining the potential of denitrification and emission of greenhouse gases, and (c) aiding in the selection of nutrient management practices for sustainable agriculture. These findings have several practical implications: (a) Incorporation of narrow C:N ratio organics (poultry and green manures) at sowing of crops could release sufficient mineral N to synchronize N supply with crop needs during early growth period, whereas some initial starter N would be needed when wide C:N ratio organics (cattle manure, pressmud, cereal crop residue) are incorporated. (b) In case of substantially enhanced immobilization of mineral N with the incorporation of wide C:N ratio crop residues, application of FN would facilitate re-mineralization after about 3-week period. (c) INM has its residual effects producing 9-35 % greater yields of succeeding crops in different cropping systems. (d) Conjoint use of legume GM and FN could alleviate the deleterious effects due to the incorporation of wide C:N ratio cereal crop residues. (f) Incorporation of groundnut crop residues in conjunction with the adequate rates of FN and FP has complementary effects in maximizing the yields, uptake of N and P, and nutrient use-efficiency in groundnut-sunflower rotation. INM enhances the yield potential of crops over and above achievable with recommended fertilizers. For example seed yield of mustard increased significantly up to 100 kg FN /ha + 30 kg P2O5/ha (which are recommended rates) but decreased thereafter with further increase in FN rate to 150 kg FN /ha due to excessive vegetative growth and resultant lodging. In contrast, all through 4 years, the combined application of GM with 100 kg N /ha further improved the yield potential of mustard by 11 %. Similar increase in the yield potential of rice (10 %) and rapeseed (16 %) in other studies illustrated the benefit that any amount of fertilizers cannot achieve.

Development of INM technologies, formulation of strategies and their adoption

These research findings led to the development of several sound INM technologies: (a) Green manuring in rice–wheat, rice–mustard, and rice–rapeseed is cost effective and economically viable. (b) Under constrained water resources, GM produced during the mild-rainy season and applied to rapeseed is more beneficial than rice-applied GM. (c) Supply of nutrients through the integrated use of 20 t GM and 60 kg FN /ha provides advantages over the use of 120 kg FN /ha alone, producing greater yields of rice and wheat while reducing the use of FN by >50 % in rice and 25 % in wheat. It significantly reduces denitrification losses and diminishes the accumulation of residual leaching to groundwater providing environmental benefits. (d) INM through GM, crop residues and FN in a rice-based cropping systems, groundnut-sunflower, soybean-based cropping systems has the long-term benefit of C sequestration and improved soil health resulting in high crop yields, help maintain balanced nutrients supply, check multinutrient deficiencies and sustain crop yields at a higher level.

Conclusions

These studies provided an insight into the practical understanding, and illustrated beyond any doubt, how INM strategy can result in agronomically feasible, economically viable and environmentally sound sustainable crop production systems by enhancing soil fertility and C sequestration, and reducing N losses and emission of greenhouse gases. Formulation and adoption of careful strategies to propagate the long-term usefulness of INM in providing nutrients and improving the soil health, educative extension efforts about the economic and environmental benefits of INM, regulations for prohibiting the burning of crop residues, and some incentives for encouraging the crop residue incorporation as a means of disposal could lead to the adoption of such eco-friendly practices.

13

Risk Management Challenges In A Changing Crop Nutrients Industry

The information and opinions contained herein are provided for informational purposes only. Any decision to purchase or sell products or commodities must be made based upon your own investigation and that of your advisors. The information contained herein is derived from sources that are believed to be reliable, but such information is not guaranteed as to accuracy or completeness. All opinions made herein may be changed at any time without notice.

Benefits of Manure and Effluent

Livestock manures are often rich in plant nutrients. Studies have shown that up to 75 percent of the nitrogen, 60 percent of the phosphorus and 80 percent of the potassium fed to dairy cattle are excreted in manure. Poultry litters and swine manures may have even higher values for phosphorus and potassium. These elements are essential plant nutrients required by all plants for normal growth and production. In addition, litter and manures contain smaller amounts of other plant nutrients including calcium, magnesium, sulfur,manganese, copper, iron, zinc, boron,molybdenum, and chloride.

Along with these nutrients,manures and litters supply valuable organic matter to help improve soil structure, soil tilth and workability, and water and nutrient holding capacities. In addition,manures and litters increase the activity of beneficial soil microbes. However,nutrient concentrations in manure can be highly variable,depending on feeding rations and methods of collection, storage and handling.

For operations using runoff and effluent containment systems, the benefits of supplemental irrigation water during periods of low rainfall are obvious. In addition, these waters will contain significant quantities of plant nutrients. However,depending on rainfall runoff amounts, effluent production and seasonal evaporational losses,nutrient concentrations vary significantly.

Soil Testing

Soil testing is the foundation of a sound fertility management program. A soil test is a series of chemical analyses on soil which estimates whether levels of essential plant nutrients are sufficient to produce a desired crop and yield. When not taken up by a crop,some nutrients, particularly nitrogen, can be lost from the soil by leaching or volatilization. Others, like phosphorus, react with soil minerals over time to form compounds which are not available for uptake by plants. Soil testing can be used to estimate how much loss has occurred and predict which nutrients and how much of that nutrients should be added to produce a particular crop and yield.

Collecting a good soil sample is the most critical step in soil testing. It is generally recommended that one "composite"soil sample be collected from each uniform area field or part of a field of 10 to 40 acres. Care should be taken to prevent sampling across areas with historically different land uses, soil types, fertilization practices, or crop yields. For fields used for routine land application of manure and wastewater, one sample per field is commonly submitted. A composite sample is obtained by combining 10 to 15 individual soil cores taken randomly across each field. The 10 cores are placed in a clean plastic bucket, thoroughly mixed and then about 1 pint is sent to the laboratory for testing. Individual soil cores can be taken using a regular spade, soil auger or soil sampling tube. First, scrape any plant residue from the surface and then make the core or boring 6 inches deep. Be careful not to remove dark colored, partially decomposed organic matter when removing plant residue. When using a spade, dig a 6-inch deep, 45 degree V-shaped hole and take a 1-inch slice from the smooth side of the hole.

Then remove a 1 by 1-inch core from the center of the shovel slice. By collecting 10 to 15 individual cores across the area, one can better ensure that the soil test results will be representative of the site and fertilizer recommendations will be appropriate. Complete sampling instructions and sample bags can be obtained from your local county Extension office.

Soil samples taken for the purpose of regulatory reporting may require more than one soil depth. For example, current regulations for most concentrated animal feed operations require composite samples from each land application field for two depths: 0 to 6 and 6 to 24 inches. Both depths should be collected at each of the 10 to 15 coring sites in a field, placed into separate buckets and submitted as separate samples to the laboratory. Care should be taken during sampling not to mix soil from the two sampling depths, to avoid obtaining incorrect results. In addition, both the sample bags and soil test information sheets should be clearly marked to distinguish between different samples and among different fields. Facilities subject to state regulations should review their permits to determine which samples and tests may be required.

Soil tests can be obtained from the Texas Agricultural Extension Service Soil,Water and Forage Testing Laboratory in College Station,Texas, or from various private laboratories across the state. Costs range from about $10 and up,depending on the laboratory and type of tests requested. typical soil test analysis. The numerical values are given in parts per million which can be multiplied by 2 to obtain estimated pounds of nutrient per acre. Depending on the crop and yield goal (as requested on the soil test information sheet), a fertilizer recommendation for all major and most minor crops in Texas will be provided by the Texas Agricultural Extension Service Soil,Water and Forage Testing Laboratory. You may need to request recommendations from many commercial laboratories.

The fertilizer recommendation can be used to determine commercial fertilizer needs, or used in conjunction with manure wastewater analyses to determine proper land application rates.

Manure and Effluent Testing

Nutrient concentrations in manures and effluents can vary substantially due to differences in feeding rations and methods of collection, handling, storage and moisture content. This will affect the fertilizer value of the material and determine proper land application rates. As a result, regular laboratory analyses of manures and effluents are strongly recommended.

In addition,annual soil testing is recommended to evaluate soil nutrient levels and adjust loading rates. To obtain samples for manure analysis, take 5 to 7 random core samples from various locations in the manure stockpile using a spade or shovel. Be certain to dig into the stockpile to collect the samples since weathering of the outside layer can change nutrient levels. Mix the core samples in a clean plastic bucket or paper bag. Place about 1 pint of the mixed sample into a sampling bag or a sealable plastic storage bag to submit for testing. Samples should be submitted as soon as possible after collection since chemical changes in the nutrients within the bag can occur during storage.

Effluent samples can be obtained by collecting 5 to 10 samples from various locations around the lagoon. These samples can be taken using a plastic bottle attached to a long pole. Mix the samples in a clean container and submit a minimum of eight ounces of the mixture in a tightly sealed plastic bottle new plastic baby bottles work well. Fill the container to within one to two inches of the top to allow for expansion. Do not use glass containers, as they may explode due to pressure buildup or break during shipment.

Topdress with additional 60 lbs/a of nitrogen after each 4 to 6 week graze down. Magnesium levels are becoming low. Consider using 150 lbs a of potassium magnesium sulfate annually. Broadcast 15 lbs of sulphur per acre. In some cases, deep rooted perennial crops may not respond to sulphur applications due to its presence in the deeper profile. Further information and assistance can be obtained from your county Extension agent:

Clearly label each sample with an identification number. This number should correspond to the one listed on the sample identification sheet submitted with the sample to the laboratory. Place all samples, information sheets and payment into a sturdy paper box for shipment to the laboratory. Keep a record of the dates and locations from which the samples were collected. Submit all samples as soon as possible after collection. Table 4 presents results from a typical laboratory analysis of manure for three samples from different sources.

Values for nitrogen, phosphorus, potassium, calcium and magnesium are given in percent (%). Multiplying these numbers by 20 will give the total pounds of nutrient per ton. For example, 1.09% nitrogen would be equivalent to 21.8 lbs N/ton. Phosphorus (P) values should then be multiplied by 2.29 to give pounds of P2O5/ton. Potassium (K) values should be multiplied by 1.2 to give pounds of K2O/ton. Other nutrients expressed in parts per million (ppm) can be multiplied by 0.002 to obtain pounds per ton.

Presents the results from a typical laboratory analysis of effluent for two samples from different sources. Values for nitrogen, phosphorus and potassium are given in percent (%). Multiply these percentages by. 2264 to obtain the total pounds of nutrient per acre-inch. Here again, phosphorus and potassium must then be multiplied by 2.29 or 1.2, respectively, to give pounds of P2O5 or K2O per acre-inch. For nutrients expressed in ppm,multiply values by 0.2264 to determine pounds per acre-inch. Manure and effluent tests can be obtained from the Texas Agricultural Extension Service Soil,Water and Forage Testing Laboratory in College Station,Texas, or from various private laboratories across the state. Costs range from about $20 and up, depending on the laboratory and type of tests requested.

Determining Land Application Rates

Land application rates should be beneficial to crops while protecting the environment. However,nutrient ratios in manures usually do not match the nutrient requirements of crops. As a result, the most efficient and economical fertilizer management strategy generally involves using a combination of manure and or effluent,and commercial fertilizer to meet crop nutrient needs. In this way, the proper balance of nutrients for optimum crop production can be provided. Phosphorus-based application rates can help prevent the buildup of phosphorus in soils. Excessive levels of phosphorus in soils can lead to nutrient imbalances which reduce crop yields, and can potentially contribute to water pollution. Once the proper application rate is determined based on soil and manure effluent testing, supplemental commercial fertilizer can be used to supply the balance of crop needs for other essential nutrients particularly nitrogen.

Management Considerations

Using manures and wastewaters effectively can greatly reduce crop fertilizer needs, and thus improve the economics of production. At the same time, application of too much manure,wastewater or commercial fertilizer, or a combination of these materials, can reduce crop yields, hurt animal performance and limit profits. When nutrients are applied at excessive rates and are not balanced with crop requirements, plant nutrient deficiencies or toxicities can occur. For example, excessive phosphorus levels in soil can cause a zinc and or iron deficiency in crops. In addition,over application and or improper spreading of manure and effluent can pollute surface and ground water with nitrates, phosphates and/or fecal bacteria. This accidental contamination of the ground and surface water can pose a health risk to you, your family and livestock,and may require years to correct.

Other best management practices which should be followed when using any fertilizer material, include:

1. Time applications of manures and fertilizers as close as possible to periods of crop nutrient need.
2. Avoid applications when the ground is frozen, saturated, or when the potential for heavy rainfall is great.
3. Inject or incorporate wastes into the soil if possible to conserve nutrients.
4. Avoid surface applications on steep (>8%) slopes.
5. Use management practices to control sediment losses.
6. Provide a filter or buffer strip (25 to 100 feet) between the application area and any nearby water resources including wells, ponds, streams, etc. (increase strip width in areas prone to erosion, slow infiltration, or limited plant growth).

Calibrating Solid Manure Spreaders

No fertilizer material can be properly applied if the rate of application is not known. A properly calibrated manure spreader will help ensure the correct amount of manure is applied.

If the size of the sheet being used is not listed, the following equation may be used to determine litter application per acre. Remember to account for the moisture content of the material if application rates are to be made on a dry weight basis. This can be done by dividing tons acre (wet weight basis) by the percent moisture content. Pounds of manure collected over sheet x 21.78 Area of sheet, ft.2 = tons acre wet weight basis To calibrate:

1. Locate a large and reasonably smooth, flat area where manure can be applied.
2. Spread the plastic sheet, tarp or bed sheet evenly on the surface of the test field.
3. Start driving the spreader at the normal application speed toward the sheet, and begin spreading at an even rate.
4. Drive over the sheet at the normal application speed while continuing to apply manure.
5. Collect all manure spread on the sheet and pour it into the bucket.
6. Weigh the bucket with manure, then subtract the weight of the empty bucket to determine pounds of manure applied to the sheet.
7. Repeat the procedure at least three times to get a reliable average.
8. Determine the average weight of the manure applications.
9. Refer to the chart in Table 6 under the appropriate sheet size to read Tons of Manure Applied Per Acre.
10. Remember to account for moisture content when determining actual land application rates on a dry weight basis.

14

Genetic Transformation of Crop Plants: Risks and Opportunities for the Rural Poor

The world population is increasing at an alarming rate and is expected to increase from 6.5 billion at present to 7.5 billion by 2025. Most of this population lives in the rural areas in the developing countries where poverty, food insecurity and nutritional deficiencies are the major problems. Low crop productivity, limited use of inputs such as fertilizers and pesticides and losses due to biotic and abiotic stress factors are a major constraint to increase production and productivity of crops. With the advent of genetic engineering, it has become possible to clone and insert genes into the crop plants to confer resistance to insect pests and improve the nutritional quality. Genetically transformed crops with Bacillus thuringiensis and herbicide resistance genes have been deployed for cultivation in USA, Canada, China and Australia. However, very little has been done to use this technology for improving crop production in the harsh environments of the tropics, where the need for increasing food production is most urgent. However, there is a need to follow the biosafety regulations and a better presentation of the results to the general public for a rational deployment of the genetically transformed crops for improving the livelihoods of the rural poor.

NEARLY 70% of poor and food-insecure people live in rural areas in the developing countries. Low productivity in agriculture is a major cause of poverty, food insecurity and poor nutrition in low-income developing countries, where agriculture is the driving force for broad-based economic growth and poverty alleviation. Productivity increases in agriculture, led by agricultural research, formed the basis of rapid economic growth and poverty reduction in many countries in Asia, Latin America and North Africa. Therefore, accelerated public investments are needed to facilitate agricultural and rural growth through high-yielding varieties resistant to biotic and abiotic stresses, environment-friendly production technology, availability of reasonably priced inputs in time, strong extension services, dissemination of information, improved infrastructure and markets, primary education, health care and adequate nutrition.

These investments need to be supported by good governance and an environment-friendly policy for sustainable management of natural resources. Advances in crop improvement have led to green revolution becoming one of the scientifically most significant events in human history. Green revolution in wheat helped to surpass in four years the production accomplishments of the past century. Land and water are diminishing resources and there is no option but to increase crop productivity per unit area. There is a need to examine how science can be used to raise biological productivity without associated ecological costs. In countries such as India, farming provides livelihood to nearly 66% of the population and there is concern that expansion of proprietary science may lead to a situation where the technologies of the future remain in the hands of a few multinational companies2. There is a genuine fear that the emerging gene revolution, spearheaded by proprietary science, can come under monopolistic control.

Therefore, there is an urgent need to take the fruits of gene revolution to the poorer sections of the society. Biotechnological approaches in agriculture and medicine can provide a powerful tool to alleviate poverty and improve the livelihoods of the rural poor. The fate of small farm families in the short-term will depend on precision agriculture, which involves the use of right inputs at the right time. Biotechnology can play an important role in integrated gene management, integrated pest management and efficient post-harvest management.

Population increase and food security

According to projections by the United Nations, world population will increase by 25% to 7.5 billion in 2020. Nearly 1.2 billion people live in a state of absolute poverty and about 800 million people are food insecure.

Food insecurity and malnutrition result in serious public health problems and a lost human potential in developing countries. The major problems faced by the rural poor include: low productivity, food insecurity and poor nutrition.

The availability of land for food production is decreasing over time and such a decrease is expected to be much greater in the developing countries than in developed countries. Mexico, Ecuador, Nigeria and Ethiopia had a per capita cropland availability of 0.25 ha in 1990 compared to below 0.10 ha in Egypt, Kenya, Bangladesh, Vietnam and China. By 2025, per capita cropland availability will be below 0.10 ha in countries such as Peru, Tanzania, Pakistan, Indonesia and the Philippines. Such a decrease in availability of cropland will have major implications for food security, particularly in the developing countries. Grain production has shown a remarkable increase from 1950 to 1980, while a marginal increase was recorded from 1980 to 1990. Thereafter, the grain production has almost remained static. The rate of increase in food production has decreased to 1% per annum in the 1990s compared to a 3% increase in the 1970s. At times people have limited access to food not because of nonavailability of food, but due to poor purchasing power. After mid-1980s, there has been a slow and steady decline in per capita availability of food grains. In India, the food production is precariously balanced despite a substantial increase in the area under irrigation. By 2001, there is a need to increase the production of pulses from 15 million tonnes in 1995 to 20 million tonnes, milk from 64 to 92 million tonnes and animal foods from 7 to 17 million tonnes. There is a general trend in reduction of number of people facing under-nutrition. The figure is expected to come down from 35% (1969–1971) to 12% in 2010. By 2010, the number of people facing malnutrition will be 30% in sub-Saharan Africa, 10% in west Asia and north Africa, 6% in east Asia, 12% in south Asia and 7% in Latin America.

The need for developing transgenic crops

One of the practical means of increasing crop production is to minimize the pest-associated losses, which are currently estimated at 14% of the total agricultural production. There are additional costs in the form of pesticides applied for pest control, currently valued at US $10 billion annually. Massive application of pesticides not only leaves harmful residues in the food, but also causes adverse effects on non-target organisms and the environment. Insect pests, diseases and weeds cause an estimated loss of US$ 243.4 billion in eight major field crops (42%), out of total attainable production of US$ 568.7 billion worldwide (Figure 2). Amongst these, insects cause an estimated loss of US$ 90.4 billion, diseases US$ 76.8 billion and weeds US$ 64.0 billion. The actual losses have been estimated at 51% in rice, 37% in wheat, 38% in maize, 41% in potato, 38% in cotton, 32% in soybean, 32% in barley and 29% in coffee. Insect pests and diseases have the potential to cause 52% loss in wheat, 58% in soybean, 59% in maize, 74% in potato, 83% in rice and 84% in cotton3. In the five most important crops of the semi-arid tropics the biotic and abiotic stress factors have been estimated to cause an estimated loss of US$ 15.74 billion.

Amongst these, the losses due to insects, diseases and weeds have been estimated to be US$ 3.17, 4.12 and 1.14 billion, respectively. Losses due to biotic stress factors have been estimated to be US$ 8.48 billion. Biotechnological approaches can be used in a rational manner to reduce the pest-associated losses in the harsh environments of the tropics. Application of pesticides to minimize the losses due to insect pests, diseases and weeds results in adverse effects on the beneficial organisms, leaves pesticide residues in the food and results in environmental pollution. As a result, chemical control of insect pests is under increasing pressure. This has necessitated the use of target-specific compounds with low persistence and an increase in emphasis on integrated pest management.

Although the benefits to agriculture from the pesticide use to prevent insect-associated losses cannot be overlooked, there is a greater need to develop alternative or additional technologies, which would allow a rational use of pesticides for sustainable crop production. Integrated pest management has historically placed great hopes on host-plant resistance. However, conventional host-plant resistance to insects involves quantitative traits at several loci and as a result, the progress has been slow and at times difficult to achieve. Many species of insect pests, plant pathogens and weeds have developed resistance to the currently available pesticides12. A large number of insects have also shown resistance to insecticides belonging to different groups and 645 cases of resistance have been documented until 1996. Maximum reports of resistance development pertain to organophosphates, followed by synthetic pyrethroids, carbamates and others including chlorinated hydrocarbons. Many species of insects have developed resistance to more than two groups of insecticides. Maximum numbers of insects and mites showing resistance to pesticides have been recorded in vegetables, followed by those infesting fruit crops, cotton cereals and ornamentals. In India, there are several documented cases of development of resistance in insects to insecticides. Maximum number of insects showing resistance to insecticides has been recorded in cotton, vegetables and tobacco. *Helicoverpa armigera* (which is the most serious pest on cotton, legumes, vegetables and cereals) has shown resistance to several groups of insecticides in cotton, tomato, chillies, sunflower, groundnut, pigeonpea and chickpea. This has resulted in widespread failure of insect control causing extreme debts, at times even forcing the farmers to commit suicide. The cotton whitefly (*Bemisia tabaci*) has shown resistance to insecticides in cotton, brinjal and okra; while tobacco caterpillar (*Spodoptera litura*) has been found to be resistant to insecticides on cotton, cauliflower, groundnut and tobacco. Green peach and potato aphid (*Myzus persicae*), cotton aphid (*Aphis gossypii*), mustard aphid (*Lipaphis erysimi*) and diamond back moth (*Plutella xylostella)* have also been found to exhibit resistance to insecticides in several crops. Development of resistance to insecticides has necessitated the application of higher dosages of the same pesticide or increased number of pesticide applications.

The farmers often resort to insecticide mixtures to minimize the insect damage to crops. This not only increases the cost of pest control, but also results in insecticidal hazards and pollution of the environment. It is in this context that the use of biotechnological techniques to contain the pest damage, both in the developed and the developing countries, becomes all the more important.

The promise of genetic engineering of crops

In addition to widening the pool of useful genes, genetic engineering also allows the use of several desirable genes in a single event and reduces the time to introgress novel genes into elite background. Research on transgenic crops, as is the case with conventional plant breeding and selection by the farmers, aims to selectively alter, add or remove a character of choice in a plant, bearing in mind the regional need and opportunities. It not only offers the possibility of bringing in a desirable character from closely-related plants, but also of adding desirable characteristics from the unrelated species. After the transformation event, the transformed plant becomes a parent for use in conventional breeding programmes.

Development and deployment of transgenic plants in an effective manner will be an important prerequisite for sustainable use of biotechnology for crop improvement. As a result of advances in genetic transformation and gene expression during the last decade13–15, there has been a rapid progress in using genetic engineering for crop improvement, of which protection of crops against the insects is a major goal. The potential of this technology has now been recognized widely. Once efficient protocols for tissue culture and transformation are developed, the production of transgenic plants with different genes is fairly routine14. Such protocols have been reported for several crops in the past.

Resistance to insect pests, diseases and herbicides

The first transgenic plants with a gene derived from *Bacillus thuringiensis* (*Bt*) were produced in 1987. While most of the insect-resistant transgenic plants have been developed by using *Bt d*-endotoxin genes, many studies are underway to use non-*Bt* genes, which interfere with the nutritional requirements of the insects. Such genes include protease inhibitors, chitinases, secondary plant metabolites and lectins. Genes conferring resistance to insects have been inserted into crop plants such as maize, cotton, potato, tobacco, rice, broccoli, lettuce, walnuts, apples, alfalfa and soybean. The first transgenic crop was grown in 1994 and large-scale cultivation was taken up in 1996 in USA. Since then, there has been a rapid growth in the area under transgenic crops in USA, Canada, Australia, Argentina and China. Successful control of cotton bollworms has been achieved through transgenic cotton.

Cry-type toxins are effective against the European corn borer and rice stem borers. Successful expression of *Bt* genes against the lepidopterous pests has also been obtained in tomato, potato, brinjal, groundnut and chickpea. Several other genes have also been deployed in the crop plants to confer resistance to insects. Transgenic plants expressing trypsin inhibitor gene have been developed in tobacco cotton and rice. Transgenic tobacco, maize and rice expressing lectin genes have shown adverse effects against several insect species feeding on these crops. Transgenic tobacco plants expressing chitinase gene have shown increased resistance to lepidopteran insects. Activity of *Bt* can also be increased in combination with tannic acid and proteinase inhibitors.

There will be tremendous benefits to the environment through the deployment of transgenic plants in pest management. Papaya ringspot virus-resistant papaya is being grown in Hawaii since 1996. Deployment of insect- resistant crops has lead to a reduction of 1 million kg of pesticides in USA44 in 1999 compared to 1998. Rice yellow mottle virus which is difficult to control with conventional approaches, can now be controlled through transgenic rice45, which would provide insurance for total crop failure. Transgenic papaya with resistance to ringspot virus46, blight resistant-potatoes and leaf blight-resistant rice48 are examples of successful control of pests through genetically modified crops.

Herbicide-resistant crops can also be used to grow crops without tillage. At the International Crops Research Institute for the Semi-Arid Tropics, several candidate genes are being evaluated for their biological efficacy against the sorghum shoot fly (*Atherigona soccata)*, spotted stem borer (*Chilo partellus)*, tobacco caterpillar (*S. litura*) and cotton bollworm or legume pod borer (*H. armigera*), which are major crop pests in the semi-arid tropics. Efforts are underway at ICRISAT to insert *Bt*, trypsin inhibitor and lectin genes into sorghum, pigeonpea and chickpea.

There has been a rapid increase in area planted to transgenic crops from 1.7 million ha in 1996 to 39.5 million ha in 1999. The value of sales has increased from US$ 0.235 billion in 1996 to US $2.3 billion in 1999. In 1997, transgenic crops were grown in 12 countries and most of the land planted to genetically improved crops was in just five countries, with USA alone accounting for about 80% of the area. Countries other than China included a number of large-scale capital-intensive farms that produce primarily for the industrial country markets. Among the crops produced in these countries are insect-resistant cotton and maize, herbicide-resistant soybean, and tomatoes with a long shelf-life. There has been a rapid increase in the area planted to herbicide- and insect-resistant crops between 1996 and 1997. Globally, herbicide-resistant soybean, insect-resistant maize and genetically improved cotton account for 85% of all plantings. Both the area planted to genetically improved crops and the value of the harvests grew dramatically between 1995 and 1999 from less than 1 million ha in 1995 to 40 million ha in 1999.

Transgenic plants with insecticidal genes are set to feature prominently in pest management in both developed and the developing world in future. Among the developing countries, China, India, Argentina, Mexico, Brazil, Pakistan and South Africa are vigorously pursuing research on transgenic crops. Entomologists, breeders, molecular biologists and agronomists need to determine how to deploy this technology for pest management and at the same time avoid or reduce possible environmental risks. To achieve these objectives, it is necessary to have an appropriate understanding of the insect biology, behaviour, its response to the insecticidal proteins, temporal and spatial expression of insecticidal proteins in the plants, strategy for resistance management and finally the impact of insecticidal proteins on natural enemies and non-target organisms.

Equally important are the issues concerning the transfer of technology to the resource-poor farmers, who will benefit greatly from these events. Biotechnology can be used for genetic transformation of the field crops for imparting resistance to the target insects and diseases, adaptation to different abiotic stress factors and improve the nutritional quality of the produce. Such an effort will play a major role in minimizing the insect-associated losses, increase crop production and improve the quality of life for the rural poor.

Improved yield

NORIN 10 genes, introduced into Western wheats in 1950s led to the green revolution in mid-sixties. These genes have now been isolated and they act in exactly the same way when used to transform other crop species. These dwarfing genes can now be deployed in other crop species to increase the productivity of different crops. Similarly, photosynthetic rates or other physiological characteristics of plants can be changed to increase the production and productivity of crops.

Tolerance to abiotic stresses

Development of crops to have inbuilt capacity to withstand abiotic stresses would help stabilize the crop production. Plants with an ability to produce more citric acid in roots, are tolerant to aluminium in acid soils A salt tolerance gene isolated from mangrove (*Avicennia marina*) has been cloned and can be transferred into other crop plants. The *gutD* gene from *Escherichia coli* can also be used to provide salt tolerance. These genes will have a great potential for use in marginal lands.

Nutritional factors

Transgenic rice, with a capacity to produce betacarotene, can be used to overcome the deficiency of vitamin A54. Transgenic rice with elevated levels of iron has been produced using genes involved in the production of an iron-binding protein that facilitates iron availability in human diet.

Pharmaceuticals and vaccines

Vaccines against infectious diseases of the gastrointestinal tract have been produced in potatoes and bananas. Anti-cancer antibodies expressed in rice and wheat can be useful in diagnosis and treatment of this disease in future. There is a great potential to increase the yield of medicines derived from plants through the use of transgenic technology.

Transgenic crops and the environment

There are a number of ecological and economic issues that need to be addressed while considering the production and deployment of transgenic crops for insect control. The most important consideration is the immediate reduction in the amount of pesticides applied for pest control. The number of pesticide applications on a crop such as cotton varies from 10 to 40 and most of the sprays are directed against the key pests such as *Helicoverpa*. In case the transgenic crops are introduced, the number of pesticide applications is likely to be reduced by two-third to half. Reduction in pesticide application would lead to an increase in the activity of the natural enemies, while some of the minor pests may tend to for the control of major pests. The magnitude of these impacts would depend on the diversity of insect species for which the crop serves as the main host. Genetically modified organisms have a better predictability of trait expression than the conventional breeding methods and the use of transgenes is not conceptually different from that of native genes or organisms modified by conventional technologies61. The potential of recombinant technologies allows a greater modification than is possible with the conventional technologies and thus might have a greater bearing on the environment.

In diverse agricultural systems such as those prevailing in the tropics, it would be important to understand the biology and behaviour of all the insect species in an ecosystem so that informed decisions can be made as to which crops to transform and the toxins to be deployed. It is also important to consider the resistance management strategies, economic value and environmental impact of the exotic genes in each crop and whether a crop serves as a source or sink for the insect pests and their natural enemies. Several studies have shown that a *Bt* toxin, which is very effective against one insect species, may be weakly active or ineffective against the other insects. Introduction of transgenic crops with insect resistance is expected to reduce the amount and number of pesticide applications. However, greater research effort is needed to identify insecticide molecules that are more effective in combination with the transgenic crops. Introduction of transgenic crops is likely to bring in a qualitative change in our approach to pest control.

The most important issues that need to be addressed while considering the deployment of transgenic crops include: (i) development of resistance, (ii) gene escape into the environment, (iii) effects on nontarget organisms and (iv) biosafety of transgenic food.

Development of resistance

Insect pest populations have a remarkable capacity to develop resistance to insecticides. Over 500 species of insects have developed resistance to insecticides. Several species of insects have shown resistance to *Bt* under laboratory and field conditions. *Bt*-resistant insect populations in Lepidoptera, Coleoptera and Diptera have been developed under laboratory conditions. In some insect species, the probability of development of resistance may be very low, e.g. *Ostrinia nubilalis*. Development of resistance to *Bt* may not be a serious issue since the *Bt* and insect pests have co-evolved for millions of years.

Gene escape into the environment

The introgression of transgenes into the wild relatives of plants is a potential concern68–70. Genes from plants engineered for herbicide resistance could cross over to other plants, creating super weeds. However, there are no records of a plant becoming a weed as a result of plant breeding. Interspecific hybridization is a common process, but hybrids are rare, and most are sterile and there is very little chance of gene introgression into the wild relatives. The possibility of movement of chloroplast from oilseed rape into wild relatives is very low. The antibiotic gene used as a marker to select for gene transfer may lead to resistance in pathogens infecting human beings. However, methods have been developed for removing selectable marker genes after selection of the transgenics. Under laboratory conditions, plasmid transfer between *B. thuringiensis* subsp. *tenebrionis* and *B. thuringiensis* subsp. *kurstali* strains occurs at a frequency of 10–2. However, no plasmid transfer has been observed in soil release experiments. A study conducted by the National Academy of Sciences, USA77 has concluded that: (i) there is no evidence of hazards associated with DNA techniques; (ii) the risks, if any, are similar to those with conventional breeding techniques; (iii) the risks involved are related to nature of the organism rather than the process; and (iv) there is a need for a planned introduction of the modified organisms into the environment.

Effects on non-target organisms

There are no significant effects of transgenic crops on the honey bees78,79. Trypsin endopeptidase inhibitor, bovine pancreatic trypsin inhibitor and soybean trypsin inhibitor have been found to be toxic to adult honey bees at 1% weight : volume in sugar solution. A few of the known predators are specialists on one insect and hence the population of the generalist predators would be maintained on the other insect species in nature. Within-field impact may be greater for parasitoids, which feed only one insect species. The populations of such natural enemies can only be maintained on the nontransgenic crops or other hosts of the target pest. The effect of transgenic crops on the abundance of natural enemies should be compared with the nontransgenic fields of the same crop where the natural enemies would be virtually absent because of heavy pesticide application.

No major differences have been observed in the abundance of predators between the transgenic and nontransgenic crops. However, two spotted ladybirds (*Adalia bipunctata*) fed for 12 days on peach–potato aphids (*Myzus persicae*) colonizing transgenic potatoes expressing lectin gene from *Galanthus nivalis* in leaves have shown a decrease in fecundity, egg viability and longevity. Increased levels of parasitism by *Campoletis sonorensis* have been observed on the transgenic plants compared to the nontransgenic plants.

Biosafety of transgenic food

The deployment of *Bt* toxin proteins in transgenic plants does not pose a health risk as the *Bt* toxins are rapidly degraded by the stomach juices of vertebrates. Rats fed on purified cowpea trypsin inhibitor have shown a moderate reduction in weight gain. Level of *G. nivalis* lectin expression that provides insecticidal protection for plants did not reduce the growth of young rats, but showed a negligible effect on weight and length of the small intestine. Therefore, careful thought should be given while considering the deployment of transgenes.

Strategies for resistance management and deployment of transgenic plants

Deployment of transgenic plants should be based on the overall philosophy of integrated pest management and should consider not only gene construct, but alternate mortality factors, reduction of selection pressure and monitor populations for resistance development to design more effective management strategies. This is particularly important when considering food security in the developing world. To increase the effectiveness and usefulness of transgenic plants, it is important to develop a strategy to minimize the rate of development of resistance in insect populations to the target genes through: (i) resistance management; (ii) gene deployment and gene pyramiding; (iii) regulation of gene expression; (iv) development of synthetics; (v) destruction of carryover population and alternate hosts; and (vi) adoption of integrated pest management strategies from the beginning.

Potential benefits of genetically transformed plants

There are many potential benefits of biotechnology for the rural poor in developing countries. Biotechnology may help achieve the productivity gains needed to feed the growing global population. It can help impart resistance to insect pests, diseases and abiotic stress factors, improve the nutritional value and enhance the durability of products during harvesting and storage. New crop varieties and biocontrol agents will reduce the reliance on synthetic pesticides and thus reduce farmers' crop protection costs, benefiting both the environment and public health. Research on genetic modification to achieve appropriate weed control will increase farm incomes and reduce the time farmers need to spend on weeding. Biotechnology would also offer cost-effective solutions to micronutrient malnutrition, such as vitamin A and iron. Research in biotechnology on increasing the efficiency of utilizing the farm input could lead to the development of crops that use water more efficiently and extract phosphate from the soil more effectively. The development of cereal plants capable of capturing nitrogen from the air could contribute greatly to plant nutrition, helping the poor farmers, who often cannot afford fertilizers. By increasing the crop productivity, agricultural biotechnology could help reduce the need to cultivate new lands and conserve biodiversity. Productivity gains could have the same poverty-reducing impact as the green revolution, if appropriate policies are put into place. There is a need to focus on crops relevant to small farmers and poor consumers in the developing countries.

There will be considerable reduction in insect damage through the deployment of transgenic crops. Transgenic maize containing *Cry 1A(b)* gene reduces the stem borer (*Diatraea* spp.) leaf feeding by 76%. However, this *Bt* toxin is largely ineffective against the fall armyworm, *Spodoptera frugiperda*. Transgenic cotton with *Bt* gene causes 94 and 91% reduction in damage in flowers and bolls, respectively. The reduction in insect damage in the transgenic crop results in 39% gain in cotton-seed yield. Analysis of the economic benefits generated by the use of herbicide-tolerant soybean seed in USA has shown that Monsanto received 22%, while seed companies gained 9% of the benefit. Consumers of soybean and soybean products in the United States and other countries shared 21% of the total benefit, while the farmers obtained 48% of the profits88. So far, development of crops has focused largely on the crops and cropping environments of North America. There is an urgent need to use biotechnological techniques to increase the productivity potential of crops that play a major role in the life of the rural poor in the developing countries. In addition to the reduction in losses due to insect pests, the development and deployment of transgenic plants with insecticidal genes will also lead to: (i) a major reduction in insecticide sprays; (ii) reduced exposure of farm labour and nontarget organisms to pesticides; (iii) increased activity of natural enemies; (iv) reduced amounts of pesticide residues in the food and food products; and (v) a safer environment to live.

Host plant resistance through the conventional breeding approaches and the transgenic crops reduces the need to apply pesticides and thus is compatible with other components of pest management in an integrated pest management programme. Pesticides are highly toxic to the natural enemies, pollinators and other nontarget organisms and result in adverse effects on the environment. Conventional HPR slows down the rate of increase of pest populations and exposes the pests for prolonged periods to the natural enemies. The introduction of transgenic plants brings in a new system of HPR into play, which has a potential to influence the tritrophic interactions87. The specificity of *Bt* is such that it was expected to have no direct effects on the natural enemies, although indirect effects such as those from the sick and sub-optimal prey would be expected. Preliminary studies have indicated that there is no adverse effect of transgenic plants on the performance of the natural enemies. However, in-depth studies need to be carried out to characterize their impact on biological control agents in the laboratory involving artificial diets and then in the field involving transgenic plants. The use of insect prediction models can further help in understanding the impact of transgenic plants on the activity and effectiveness of natural enemies in controlling insect pests in conjunction with the transgenic crops.

Limitations

Transgenics are not a panacea for solving all the pest problems. There are some genuine or perceived concerns. The major limitations of transgenic plants are:

- Secondary pests are not controlled in the absence of sprays for the major pests.
- Need to control the secondary pests through chemical sprays will kill the natural enemies and thus offset one of the advantages of transgenic crops.
- Proximity to sprayed fields and insect migration may reduce the benefits of transgenic crops.

Development of resistance in insect populations may limit the usefulness of transgenic crops.

There is a considerable debate about the risks such as development of resistance in insect pests to *Bt* toxins, harmful effects on beneficial insects and crosspollination of wild and weedy plants with the novel gene. The evidence on these issues is still inconclusive and warrants careful monitoring before the transgenic crops are deployed on a large scale. The biggest risk of modern biotechnology for developing countries is that technological development may bypass poor farmers because of a lack of enlightened adaptation. It is not that biotechnology is irrelevant, but research needs to focus on the problems of small farmers in developing countries. Private sector research is unlikely to give priority to such crops, given the lack of future profits.

Without a stronger public sector role, a form of scientific apartheid may develop, in which cutting-edge science becomes exclusively oriented towards industrial countries and large-scale farming. Successful adoption of green revolution technologies depended largely on access to water, fertilizers and pesticides. As a result, inequality between well-endowed and resource-poor farmers increased because of the properties of the technology itself. Excessive and improper use of chemical inputs also led to adverse environmental impact. A major ethical concern is that genetic engineering and life patents accelerate the reduction of plants, animals and micro-organisms to mere commercial commodities. Therefore, all agricultural activities that constitute human intervention into natural systems and processes need to be assessed carefully.

Regulations for production and release of transgenic plants

The permission for release of modified organisms is given after the risk assessment by the individual countries Some initiatives have already been taken in this direction by NAS in USA91 and OECD. International organizations such as UNIDO, UNEP, FAO and WHO have published a voluntary code of conduct for release of organisms into the environment.

Regulations for handling and release of genetically modified plants in India

The Department of Biotechnology, Ministry of Science and Technology, Government of India, has formulated guidelines in 1986 for the release of DNA in 1990 under the Environmental Protection Act. These include institutional biosafety committees to monitor the research activities at the institute level, review committee on genetic manipulation functioning in the DBT and genetic engineering approval committee of the Ministry of Environment and Forests, that has the authority to permit large-scale use of transgenics at the commercial level. The DBT has set up the rDNA committee to prepare modified draft of guidelines from time to time on the basis of current scientific information and from the experience gained locally and outside the country. In general, the biosafety guidelines deal with the definition of rDNA, classification of pathogenic micro-organisms, containment facilities, biosafety levels, rDNA research activities, large-scale experiments, release of transgenics, import and shipment of rDNA and its products and quality of biological materials produced through rDNA technology.

Risk assessment for the deployment of transgenic plants

There is need for a thorough investigation regarding the fate of modified organisms in the environment and their interaction with the wild relatives and the nontarget organisms. Genetically engineered crops can play an important role in pest management and reduce the amount of pesticide applied for pest control, thus leading to reduction of pesticide residues in food and resulting in conservation of the environment. Therefore, it may be important to go beyond the immediate considerations of their influence on the environment. Production and release of transgenic plants should be based on experience and there is a need to streamline and harmonize the regulatory requirements for deployment of genetically engineered micro-organisms and plants for pest management. The promise of biotechnology for increasing the production and productivity of crops for sustainable crop production has been dimmed by the intrinsic safety of the transgenic organisms and evolution of resistant strains of insects. Social and environmental groups have raised a hue and cry about the real conjectural effects on the nontarget organisms. In the developed countries, biotechnology is seen to be of strategic importance for increasing the share of world market. However, there are serious concerns about the introduction of this technology in several countries. The focus of biosafety regulations should be on safety, quality and efficacy. Data required for risk assessment include (i) organization and the people involved; (ii) DNA donor, the receiving species, and the transgenic plant; (iii) target environment and the conditions of release; (iv) transgenic plant and environment interaction; and (v) monitoring, control and waste treatment. General information includes the institution and the people involved in development and the people organizations to be responsible for field containment, monitoring and waste treatment. DNA donor and receiving species include complete information about the donor and the receiving species. Information is also needed on the vector and antibiotic or herbicide resistance genes used as a marker. The receiving plant species forms the baseline with which the transgenic plant should be compared. The risk to the environment includes harmful effects on the beneficial nontarget organisms.

It is important to describe the invasiveness of the transgenic plant in the wild habitat, ability to propagate sexually/asexually, possibility of transferring the transgene to the same or related species or to microorganisms and the consequences of gene transfer. Once the transgenic plants are released into the environment, there is a free movement of pollen, seed and the plants outside the immediate environment of release. It is important to monitor the transgenes in the environment after the release and the efficiency with which it is possible to destroy the plant material. Detection of the transgenic plants and the transgene in the nontarget species can be done by visual markers (e.g. *b*- glucorinidase) or a selectable marker (e.g. antibiotic resistance or molecular analysis, e.g. PCR and Southern hybridization). The following issues need to be addressed while considering the deployment of transgenic plants:

- Care should be taken that the release of transgenic plants does not give rise to new pest problems or emergence of new biotypes of the target pest and whether the transgenic technology possess greater risk than the traditional alternatives.
- In case of gene transfer to the wild relatives, will it lead to expansion of the niche of the species and result in suppression of diversity in the surrounding areas?
- Will the introduction of transgenic plant result in an increase in the land use for agriculture, where agriculture could not be practised earlier, i.e. bringing valuable natural ecosystem under agriculture?

The risk assessment should be standardized for the plants new to the environment. Most nations already have procedures for development and release of new crop varieties. Although these procedures were primarily based on agronomic performance, the same can be used as a model for a more formal risk assessment to investigate the potential environmental impact of transgenic plants. In world agriculture, if the developing countries have to benefit from the transgenic technology, it is important to promote capacity building and risk management including: (i) scientific and technical team research; (ii) strengthen the infrastructure; (iii) monitor short- and long-term effects of transgenic plants; and (v) develop simple techniques to distinguish transgenic and nontransgenic plants.

Socio-economic issues and biotechnology

Genetic homogeneity enhances genetic vulnerability to biotic and abiotic stresses. Biotechnology companies are therefore recommending resistance management strategies, such as growing 30 to 40% non-*Bt* corn with *Bt*-corn. This has serious implications for the livelihood of small and marginal farmers operating with institutional credit. If transgenic crops are affected by serious diseases as a result of the breakdown of resistance, there will be a catastrophic effect on the lives of poor farmers. The companies will have to agree to compensate them for the crop loss. This problem could become even more serious if companies incorporate genetic use restriction mechanisms, popularly known as 'terminator gene' in the new crop varieties. Farmers will have to purchase the new seeds each year. The other dimension is equity in benefit sharing between biotechnologists and the primary conservers of genetic resources and the holders of traditional knowledge. The primary conservers have so far remained poor, while those who use their knowledge (for example, the medicinal properties of plants) and material have become rich. This has resulted in accusations of biopiracy. It is time that molecular biologists and others find ways to implement genuine biopartnerships with the holders of indigenous knowledge and traditional conservers of genetic variability, based on principles of ethics and equity in benefit sharing.

Unless research and development efforts on transgenics are based on principles of bio-ethics, there will be serious public concerns about the ultimate nutritional, social, ecological and economic consequences of replacing local varieties with a few, new genetically improved crop varieties. Bulk of modern agricultural biotechnology research is undertaken by the private sector, which protects intellectual property rights (IPR) through patents that extend beyond the first release of transgenic crops. Farmers, therefore, cannot legally plant or sell the seed of patented cultivars without the consent of the patent holder. However, monitoring and enforcing contracts that prohibit large numbers of small farmers from using the crops they produce as seed would be expensive and difficult.

Public perceptions about biotechnology are not based on fact and there is a tendency to over-emphasize the risks to gain public attention59. Also there is a risk of modern science bypassing the needs of rural poor as a result of the patenting regime adopted by the multinational companies and the negative role played by the environmental groups. Research in progressive biotechnology should be integrated with appropriate policies and conventional breeding. The benefits and the risks associated with the use of biotechnology to increase agricultural production need to be presented to the general public in a balanced manner and concern for moral and ethical issues of relevance to different societies need to be addressed. Public trust in the application of biotechnology for increasing and stabilizing agricultural production needs to be improved to use modern science for the benefit of the rural poor.

Future outlook

The use of crop protection traits through transgenics will continue to expand in future and gene pyramiding will become very common, which may be related to genetic transformation with two or more genes against the same trait or different traits. There will be considerable emphasis on agronomic traits such as fertilizer-use efficiency, stress tolerance, photosynthetic efficiency and grain yield and quality. This approach of controlling insect pests and diseases would offer the advantage of allowing some degree of selection for specificity effects, so that pests, and not the beneficial organisms are targeted. Research on agricultural biotechnology can contribute to food security in developing countries provided it focuses on the needs of poor farmers and consumers.

It is also important that biotechnology be viewed as a component of comprehensive poverty alleviation and it needs to go hand in hand with investment programme in agricultural growth. Public sector research, particularly through partnerships between the International Agricultural Research Centres and National Agricultural Research Systems, is essential for ensuring that molecular biology-based science serves the needs of the rural poor. It is important that internationally-accepted biosafety standards and local regulatory capacity be strengthened within developing countries. Open debate about the issues involved is essential to present the benefits and the risks associated with the deployment of transgenic crops to the general public in a balanced manner. If appropriate steps are not taken, modern biotechnology could bypass poor people and opportunities for reducing poverty, food insecurity and malnutrition will be missed. Hence, it is important to undertake urgent steps to use biotechnology for improving the livelihood of the rural poor.

15

Mineral Nutrition of Fruit Crops

In addition to water, sunlight, and carbon dioxide from the air, plants require 13 mineral nutrients that are typically derived from the soil. The macronutrients nitrogen (N), phosphorus (P), potassium (K) are needed by plants in relatively large amounts and often have to be added to the soil. Intermediate amounts of secondary nutrients magnesium (Mg), calcium (Ca), and sulfur (S) are needed by plants. Trace or micronutrients [boron (B), chlorine (Cl), copper (Cu), iron (Fe), manganese (Mn), molybdenum (Mo) and zinc (Zn)] are needed in small amounts and are seldom deficient in Wisconsin soils.

In a healthy plant the essential mineral elements are present in adequate levels and in correct proportion to other elements. Plant productivity or fruit quality is reduced if:

- One or more of the required elements is not present in sufficient quantity (deficiency);
- One or more elements is present in too great a quantity (toxicity);
- Or the levels of one or more elements is out of balance with other nutrients.

These nutrients perform a variety of functions in plants ranging from being structural components of cell walls and membranes to activating enzyme systems. About 95% of the dry weight of a typical plant is made up of carbon, oxygen and hydrogen. The soil supplied minerals make up only 5% of a plants total dry weight.

The nutrition of plants and animals is very different. While animals need proteins, carbohydrates, vitamins and minerals to be healthy, plants need only water, sunlight and the 13 essential nutrients. No scientific evidence supports the use of vitamins or other similar supplements for plant growth. Plants don't need to be "fed". They simply need adequate supplies of water, sunlight and minerals. While fertilizers can be added to soils to improve their fertility, the best plan is to establish your fruit planting on a fertile soil. The soil pH should be between 6 and 7 for optimum production. Ag limestone must be incorporated to be effective because lime only moves about ½ inch per year if topdressed. Plants can make best use of soil applied nutrients if these nutrients are distributed within the soil rooting volume.

Factors affecting soil fertility

Soil fertility is a complex concept referring to the potential of a soil to supply nutrients in amounts, forms and proportions required for optimum plant growth. Describing soil fertility in detail is beyond the scope of this bulletin. Soil properties that affect the nutrient supply to plants include cation exchange capacity, soil pH and soil texture.

Cation Exchange Capicity

One of the most important "reservoirs" of plant nutrients in the soil is the exchangeable nutrients held on cation exchange sites. Most of the potassium, ammonium, calcium and magnesium used by plants comes from the exchange sites. Each soil has a finite capacity to hold positively charged nutrients, the cation exchange capacity. Silty and clayey soils can hold several times more positively charged nutrients than sandy soils. However, even sands have adequate exchange capacity to hold all of the nutrients needed by plants in an available form.

Soil pH

Establishing and maintaining proper soil pH by use of ag limestone plays an important role in productivity because of the influence soil pH has on nutrient availability and other chemical biological processes affecting plant growth. Soil pH affects the availability of plant nutrients. Optimum availability of plant essential nutrients is ensured if mineral soil pH is maintained between 6.0 and 6.5 (except for blueberries and other *Vaccinium*). In some instances nutrient deficiencies or toxicities can be avoided by adjusting soil pH to the proper level.

Organic Matter

Soil organic matter affects both the chemical and physical properties of a soil even though it makes up only 1 to 5 percent of the soil mass. In addition to holding available plant nutrients in an exchangeable form, organic matter releases nutrients when it decomposes. Crop residues, manure, and other organic materials contain significant amounts of nitrogen, phosphorus, sulfur and boron and serves as a "reservoir" for these nutrients, which become available as soil microorganisms convert the organic nutrients into inorganic, plant available forms.

Soil organic matter influences soil physical characteristics such as soil erosion, soil temperature, water holding capacity and drainage. Additions of organic materials will increase the amount of water held available for crops in sandy soils and improve drainage in heavier textured soils by its influence on pore space. Adding organic matter to soils as manure or green manure crops before planting is more beneficial than surface applications with no incorporation after plant establishment

Texture

Soil texture describes the feel of the soil, its coarseness or fineness. More specifically it is the relative proportion of sand, silt and clay that make up the mineral portion of a soil. All textures of soil are found in various parts of Wisconsin. Fruit will grow in most soil types as long as they have enough, but not too much, water and nutrients. Additions of organic matter will help minimize soil limitations due to texture but will not entirely alleviate severe problems.

Plant response and soil fertility

Soil fertility can be thought of as the ability of the soil to supply nutrients needed for optimum yield. A soil test is the most practical way of measuring the nutrient supplying power of the soil and telling if fertilizer and/or lime are needed.

Fertilizers are applied to supply essential nutrients that may be in short supply or unavailable to plants from the soil. Plants absorb nutrients from the soil and use them to produce new growth or fruit. The application of agricultural fertilizers has greatly increased crop yields over the past 50 years by eliminating nutrient availability as a major limitation to yield.

When a particular nutrient is in short supply, application of additional nutrient will increase growth and yields. Initially this may be a linear response where yield increases one unit per unit of fertilizer added. At some point the response levels out and yield increases become less pronounced as additional fertilizer is applied. This is followed by a plateau where yield is not increased with additional applications of nutrients. However, plants may continue to absorb nutrients without having a corresponding increase in yields. This is known as luxury consumption. At the far end of the plateau there is a point where excessive nutrient levels, especially micronutrients, may become toxic to plants and will reduce yields. The goal in applying fertilizer is to supply enough nutrients to provide optimal plant growth without supplying too much fertilizer.

Diagnosing the mineral nutrition status of fruit crops

Fruit growers have three main tools to use in evaluating the mineral nutrition status of their plantings. These are:

- Examine visual symptoms exhibited by leaves, stems, and fruit;

- Aalyzing leaf tissue and;
- Testing the soil.

Used together properly these are powerful tools that can be used to prevent nutrient deficiencies or toxicities as well as to assess current fertility management practices.

Visual Symptoms

Visual symptoms have been used for many years to diagnose deficiencies of certain elements. Color photographs of various deficiency symptoms have been published as diagnostic tools. However, there are at least two disadvantages associated with this approach as the primary method for estimating nutrient need. First, once the visual symptoms have appeared the crop quality and yield has likely already been reduced. Second, some visual deficiency symptoms look similar while others may be confused with disease, insect or environmental stress symptoms. Further confusion arises when the symptoms from more than one deficient element is confounded by a deficiency or toxicity of another.

Tissue Analysis

Tissue analysis is a powerful tool in assessing mineral nutrition of crops. Chemically analyzing the concentration of nutrients in the leaves of growing crops can more precisely define the nutrient status than an examination of deficiency symptoms. This is particularly true for perennial fruit crops. This method is based on collecting samples of tissue in the field and measuring the amounts of mineral elements in the tissue. Tissue analysis provides a "snapshot" picture of the nutrient status of a crop at a particular point in time resulting from all factors that affect plant growth. In addition to confirming suspected deficiencies, plant analysis can also detect toxicities or hidden deficiencies before visual symptoms appear. Experimentation has shown the amounts of the various minerals that should be present in plants to provide optimal growth. These amounts are different for each crop species.

Collecting a sample

The most important part of tissue analysis is taking a proper sample. Nutrient levels within plants differ depending on the plant part sampled, the stage of maturity, the location on the plant and environmental factors. It is important to follow standard sampling procedures for each fruit crop. Plants must be sampled at the proper stage of maturity in order to correctly interpret the results. Nitrogen, for example, is relatively high in leaves in the spring, levels off in midseason and then declines in the late summer and fall before the leaves drop. Interpretations are based on knowing the relationship between nutrient levels in a particular part of a "standard" tissue in a specific time in the growing season. A leaf sample taken in the spring could show excess nitrogen compared to mid season standards and a sample taken in the fall could show a deficiency even if it were adequate at mid season. Samples taken at a time during the season different than the "standards" used for nutrient interpretation will likely show erroneous results.

Sampling a different plant part than the "standards" will also lead to incorrect interpretations of the analysis. For example, nitrogen is mobile in plants and old leaves are the first to show deficiency symptoms. If old leaves are sampled a deficiency may be indicated, while if young leaves are sampled an adequate amount or an excess may be shown. The correct plant part to sample. The sample should be representative of the planting because the results of the test can be no better than the sample sent in for analysis. The amount of tissue the lab actually tests is less than a teaspoon, so it is very important that the sample be characteristic of the field or block. If the planting consists of different cultivars that are intermixed, take leaves from each cultivar. Make sure an adequate number of plants are sampled. Don't sample diseased, damaged, insect infested or abnormal tissue. If you suspect a nutrient related disorder, sample early in the growing season. Submit a sample of abnormal appearing tissue along with a sample not showing the symptoms that is collected on the same day. By doing so a comparison of the two samples can be made and a better evaluation can be made between the nutritional status of healthy and abnormal plants. Include a soil sample with your plant analysis sample. Soil test results for pH, organic matter, and available P and K can be useful when interpreting the plant tissue results. In Wisconsin, a routine soil analysis is included as part of the plant analysis program at no additional cost.

Submitting a sample

Once the tissue sample has been collected it should be prepared for shipment or delivery to the lab. Any soil or foreign material should be dusted off the sample. DO NOT WASH the leaves as this will remove soluble nutrients. If the sample is to be mailed, allow the sample to air dry for one day to prevent mold from forming during shipment. Place the dry sample in a paper envelope for shipping. Do not use plastic or cellophane bags since these retain moisture and promote molding. Try to ship samples early in the week (Wednesday at the latest) to avoid samples deteriorating in warm post offices over the weekend. Plant samples that are delivered to the lab do not need to be air dried if they are delivered within a day after sampling. Please submit an information sheet describing the crop type, date sampled, and other information necessary to make the best interpretations of lab results. Plant analysis information sheets are available from the laboratory or your County Extension office.

Soil analysis

Soil testing is a means of measuring soil pH and estimating the supply of nutrients available for plant growth. There is a poor relationship between soil and plant nutrient levels in perennial fruit crops, particularly tree fruits. When plant tissue levels from tissue analysis are compared to corresponding soil nutrient contents from soil analysis, no correlation is found. Therefore, soil testing alone may not provide enough information to make accurate fertilizer decisions for perennial fruit crops. Reliable commercial soil tests have not been developed for nitrogen, copper or iron. The need for these elements can best be evaluated by plant analysis. Deficiencies of most minor elements can better be identified by plant analysis too. Some fertility problems such as those associated with very acid or very alkaline soils are difficult to identify by plant analysis alone and are better evaluated by a soil test when used in concert with tissue analysis.

Soil testing

Soil samples should be taken from the same areas as the tissue samples. For strawberries, raspberries and grapes take the sample to the side of the plant row, but not in the middle between the rows. For tree fruits take the sample within the drip line of a tree and within the vegetation free area. Don't sample from the sod area.

Take individual samples with a trowel or small shovel. A good sample consists of about 8-10 subsamples, taken to 6 inches, per area. Mix the subsamples and place about 1 cup of soil in a soil bag or pint plastic bag. Identify the bag with the same sample number as the corresponding tissue sample. Submit the soil sample along with the tissue sample for analysis to the lab of your choice. Be sure the bags are sealed tightly so the tissue samples cannot be contaminated with soil. No fee is assessed for routine soil analysis corresponding with a tissue sample at the UWEX lab. A soil analysis should always be a part of preparing the site before planting. Because fruit plants are relatively long lived it makes sense to amend the soil prior to planting. Take soil samples from the site a year before planting and apply and deeply incorporate any fertilizer or lime recommended. This is an especially good practice for strawberries since they are replanted every 3 to 5 years. A soil test is the only practical means to determine which and how much fertilizer andor lime are needed for best growth. Evaluating soil fertility is a good practice to establish in order to make most efficient use of applied fertilizer.

Interpreting the report

About two weeks after samples have been submitted you will receive a computerized report showing the concentrations of various nutrients in the tissue and soil. Beside each number is a letter designation indicating that the concentration is deficient, low, sufficient, high or in excess for that nutrient. This interpretation is provided only if the plant was sampled at the proper stage of maturity. Soil pH, organic matter and an estimate of plant available phosphorus and potassium will also be reported if a soil sample was submitted. If soil was not sampled, interpretations of plant tissue results will be based on an assumption of optimum soil test results.

The indication that the tissue nutrient concentration is deficient, low, adequate, high or excessive will tell you whether applications of fertilizer program is warranted. Long experience and experimentation has shown what concentrations of each required element should be found in plant tissues. Interpretation of the results with these standards is possible only if the correct plant part was sampled at the proper stage of maturity. No valid interpretation is possible if the wrong part was sampled or the plants are sampled at other times in the season.

Fertilizer application

Fertilizers are materials that contain nutrients required by plants. In some cases, organic materials such as manures and plant residues can supply some or all the nutrients required by plants. However, plants cannot differentiate between nutrients from organic, inorganic, liquid or granular sources. All nutrients are absorbed by plant roots as ions and all ions of a given element are identical regardless of the source. The benefits from using organic materials on soils are many, but relate mostly to 1) the contribution of mobile nutrients (nitrogen) in a slowly available form and 2) improvement of the physical condition of the soil. Since plant nutrient requirements can be met with easily blended and precisely measured commercial fertilizers, the use of organic materials is encouraged mostly for their beneficial effect on soil physical properties. Fertilizers can be applied to the soil and taken up by the roots or applied to the plant as a liquid for uptake by the leaves, stems or fruit. Each method has advantages. Soil application is usually less expensive and is better suited for large application rates of the major nutrients and for pre-plant application. For the most part, soil applications by broadcasting, banding or top dressing are the most economical and efficient.

Foliar application is best for correcting micronutrient deficiencies or for increasing the concentration of immobile elements to specific tissues, such as calcium and boron to fruits and flower buds, respectively. Liquid fertilizers that are foliar applied are more expensive per unit of nutrient. In many cases the liquid fertilizer runs off, or is washed off leaves onto the soil where it is later taken up by the roots. In this case it would have been much less expensive to apply a granular fertilizer to the soil. The expense of foliar applications of nutrients may be decreased if they can be mixed with pesticides in a cover spray. Fertilizers commonly used on fruit crops are described below.

Fertilizers

A soil and or plant tissue analysis are the most reliable methods to determine nutrient need and amount. Nutrients of most common concern to Wisconsin growers include nitrogen, phosphorus, potassium, calcium, boron and zinc.

Nitrogen

Nitrogen is the nutrient most commonly applied to fruit crops. It is usually applied in one of two inorganic forms: ammonium or nitrate. Research comparing these two forms of nitrogen have shown each to be equally effective in supplying nitrogen to most fruit crops, however, cranberries and blueberries use only ammonium nitrogen. Nitrogen may also be applied in organic forms as manures, fish hydrolysate, mulches, etc. The timing of nitrogen fertilizer applications can affect their efficiency and potential for losses. Sources that are least expensive per unit of nitrogen are preferred.

Phosphate

Wisconsin soils typically contain enough phosphate to

supply plant needs. An average fruit crop would remove only 6 to 12 pounds of phosphate per acre per year. This amount does not need to be applied annually. As phosphate is removed from the soil solution by plants, additional previously insoluble phosphorus moves into the soil solution to maintain an equilibrium. This phosphorus is available because it binds tightly to the soil matrix in a plant available but relatively immobile form.

The best time to add phosphate fertilizer is before the crop is planted. Based on a preplant soil test, the soil should contain 25 ppm soil test phosphorus. Once plants are in the ground it is difficult to incorporate phosphate fertilizer into the rooting zone. Maintaining soil pH between 6 and 6.5 will ensure maximum availability of soil phosphorus. All commonly used phosphate fertilizers presently sold in Wisconsin (except rock phosphate) contain at least 85% water soluble phosphorus. Rock phosphate is not an effective phosphorus source for most Wisconsin soils.

Potassium

Fruit crops are relatively heavy potassium users. Some Wisconsin soils will require additions of applied potassium because of removal by crops and because Wisconsin soils have little native exchangeable potassium. A typical acre of soil may contain 20,000 ppm of total potassium in the top 6 inches, but nearly all of this is a structural component of soil minerals and is unavailable to plants. Plants can only use the exchangeable potassium on the surface of soil particles and the potassium dissolved in soil solution. A soil test measures the readily available form of potassium in soil. Tissue testing is critical to monitoring potassium levels. A fruit crop may remove 20 to 40 pounds per acre of potash per year. Potassium deficiency can be exacerbated by high tissue nitrogen or low soil moisture.

Potassium fertilizer is best added to soils and incorporated before the crop is planted. Soil test levels of about 100 ppm (200 lbs/A), depending on soil type, are recommended. If tissue or soil samples show low potassium levels, it should be corrected as soon as possible. In areas where potassium deficiency is a problem annual applications of potash may be warranted, depending on the crop and soil type. If soil potassium levels are high, less potash fertilizer is needed allowing for some decrease in soil test level.

Calcium

Calcium is critical for the growth of quality fruit It binds cell walls together and helps maintain fruit firmness. Bitter pit and cork spot are physiological disorders of apple that are calcium related. Wisconsin soils typically contain adequate amounts of calcium. However, adequate amounts of calcium may not reach developing fruit. Calcium is relatively immobile in plants and developing fruit are not able to draw calcium from adjacent tissues. Calcium deficiency can be exacerbated by high nitrogen and low soil moisture.

Calcium is the predominant positively charged ion held on soil and organic matter surfaces. Leaching of calcium does not occur to any appreciable extent because of its relatively strong attraction to the soil. The relationship between tissue test calcium and flower bud or fruit calcium is not very strong. Even if tissue levels of calcium are sufficient, fruit may be deficient.

Calcium moves into tissues through the xylem in the transpiration stream. Since fruit don't lose a lot of water through evaporation, not enough calcium may flow to the fruit. Some apple cultivars are more susceptible to calcium related disorders than others. A history of calcium related fruit disorders is good evidence that additional calcium is needed. Applying calcium to the soil has not been an effective fertilizer practice to increase leaf or fruit calcium concentrations. Soil limed to pH 6-6.5 has more than adequate levels of available calcium for fruit crops. The problem is in moving calcium to the developing fruit. To improve fruit calcium content, calcium can be applied directly to the fruit and absorbed through the skin. Calcium chloride is the least expensive form of calcium that can be applied to fruit plants to increase tissue calcium. Calcium chloride is very corrosive to metal so spray equipment should be cleaned thoroughly after application. Calcium chloride can build up on leaves and cause leaf burning. Repeat applications should not be made unless rain has been received since the last application. The recommended application regime for apples is to add calcium chloride to cover sprays beginning with the first cover spray (early June) at the rate of 2 lbs per 100 gallons dilute or 4 lbs per acre concentrate. This can be increased to 3 lbs per 100 gallons and 6 lbs per acre concentrate for later sprays. Calcium chloride is compatible with most pesticides and should not alter their action nor affect fruit finish. Three or four applications per year should be sufficient to increase fruit calcium content. Calcium sprays will not eliminate calcium related disorders, but should reduce their incidence.

Boron

Boron is the micronutrient that is most likely to be deficient in fruit plantings in the Midwest. Soils may contain 0.5 to 2.0 ppm of available boron, but more that 5.0 ppm available boron can be toxic to many crops. Most of the boron in soils is in the organic matter. As a result, most of the available boron is in the plow layer where organic matter is highest. Soils low in organic matter are deficient in boron more often than soils with high organic matter content. Soils with a pH of 7.0 or above are more likely to be deficient in boron than are more acidic soils.

Boron is essential to proper flower development and pollen germination. Although required in small amounts its role is very critical and deficiencies may reduce yields severely. Minor deficiencies can be corrected by soil application of boron containing fertilizers. Severe deficiencies can be mitigated by foliar application. The most common boron fertilizers are borax and sodium tetraborate. Solubor, sodium pentaborate and boric acid are used occasionally for soil application or in a foliar spray. Foliar boron is usually applied as a soluble 20.5% wettable powder applied at 2.5 lbs per acre or 10 ounces per

100 gallons dilute. Do not apply over 5 lbs of boron per acre per year as toxicity may occur. Soil application can be made at any convenient time during the year. Foliar application should be made in the fall after harvest but while the leaves are still green and active or in the spring at the pink stage of flower development.

Organic fertilizers

Nutrients can also be applied in organic forms such as manures, compost, mulches, etc. These materials have the added advantage of adding organic material to the soil which will help maintain soil structure, improve water holding capacity and drainage characteristics. Composts and mulches have relatively little nutrient value. These are usually considered soil conditioners, and credit is usually not given to their minimal nutrient content. However, sometimes organic materials such as manure cannot supply all of the nutrients needed by plants in sufficient quantities to optimize yields.

Supplementing organic fertilizers with synthetic fertilizers may be necessary for best management of applied nutrients and optimum yields. Organic fertilizers are, by their very nature, highly variable in their nutrient content.

Summary

Fertility of fruit crops is an important management practice where much misinformation exists. Plants require light, water and 13 mineral elements to grow and produce fruit. Growers need to be sure that these needs are met. Once you provide an adequate nutrient supply, additional nutrient applications will not enhance yields, only reduce profits. You can monitor the nutrient status of your fruit crop by routine soil and tissue analysis. By doing so, you can prevent deficiencies before they occur and minimize inefficient use of applied nutrients.

16

Nutrient Resources for Crop Production in the Tropics

For the foreseeable future a majority of the population, and almost all the mal- and under-nourished, will continue to be found in the tropics and subtropics. Food security in these parts of the world will have to be met largely from local resources. The productivity of the land is to a large extent determined by the fertility of the soil, which in turn is mostly determined by its organic matter content and stored nutrients. Soil organic matter is readily lost when organic matter inputs are reduced upon cultivation and more so upon intensification. The concomitant loss of topsoil and possible exposure of subsoil acidity may cause further soil degradation.

With current urban expansion, nutrients in harvested products are increasingly lost from the rural environment as a whole. Estimates of soil nutrient depletion rates for sub-Saharan Africa are alarmingly high. The situation may be more favourable in Latin America and Asia where fertilizer inputs are tenfold those of SSA. Closing the nutrient cycle at a community level in rural areas may be tedious; on an inter-regional level it is associated with considerable costs of collection, detoxification and transportation to the farms. Yet, at the rate at which some of the non-renewable resources such as phosphorus and potassium are being exploited, recycling of these nutrients will soon be required.

Nutrient Requirements and Supplies

The productivity of the soil is largely determined by its fertility, which in turn is dependent on rootable soil depth and the nutrients stored in its mineral and organic constituents. The rootable soil depth may be restricted by physical constraints such as water table, bedrock or other impenetrable layers, as well as by chemical problems such as soil acidity, sodicity, salinity or toxic substances. Large reserves of stored nutrients are in themselves no guarantee of high soil fertility as plant availability of nutrients requires the release of these nutrients from their mineral or organic matrix or surfaces, processes that can be physical, chemical, as well as biological in nature. Finally, a fertile soil can be of benefit to the plant only in the presence of sufficient soil water to allow the transport of these nutrients to the plant's roots.

Loss of soil productivity is often related to the loss of soil organic matter, which not only leads to a reduction in soil fertility, but also in the structure, water holding capacity and biological activity of a soil. Soil organic matter is readily lost when organic matter inputs are reduced upon cultivation, and this occurs more rapidly under tropical conditions. Jenny & Raychaudhuri studied 522 soils in India and calculated the percentage loss of SOM as a result of cultivation. They found carbon losses ranging from near 0% for paddy soils up to around 70% for the most fragile environments. Organic nitrogen followed a similar trend. The introduction of intensive agriculture with its reliance on NPK fertilizers has placed inordinate demands on the soil to provide the remaining essential nutrients. Moreover, in many developing countries fertilizer use favours nitrogen disproportionately to the crops' demands. As a result, the long-term use of chemical fertilizers may disturb soil nutrient balances or cause soil acidification. Thus, intensive agriculture may have amplified the magnitude and increased the rate of the age-old problem of soil degradation.

Agro-Ecosystem Differentiation

Nutrient requirements are widely different and dependent on the crop and the production potential of the environment. The natural vegetation often re¯ects the constraints to primary production of that environment such as proneness to drought, excess water or heat, soil acidity or salinity. It is tempting to infer nutrient requirements of an agro-ecosystem from biomass produced by its natural vegetation, but this often leads to the wrong conclusions as it overlooks the time factor involved in arriving at this biomass. Moreover, human interference often changes the system from one with a closed nutrient cycle to one that is more or less open, depending on the severity of the human impact, with the resulting degradation of the resource base discussed above. Conversely, human intervention may overcome most soil constraints, but often only at a considerable, sometimes prohibitive cost. As a result, the production potential may vary in space and time. The costs associated with soil fertility improvement are a function of the expected resulting outputs and vary from region to region. The differentials in these costs lead to different strategies to satisfy plant nutrient demands.

Traditional agriculture

The area of the eastern Amazon of Brazil, known as the Bragantina region, was colonized some 100 years ago and has since been converted from a primary forest region to a natural forest±fallow cultivation system. Slashing and burning has been used traditionally to prepare the land for the 1±2 year cultivation phase. With increasingly shorter fallow cycles, approaching 3±7 years instead of the traditional 15±25 years, the productivity of the system has gradually diminished, attributable in large part to the loss of nutrients from the system. The problem is common to many moist tropical forest areas and has been given ample attention in the literature. A rather extensive research programme in the area has allowed a preliminary assessment of the nutrient budgets in this system.

In the current land use cycle with about seven years fallow, yields of maize, cowpea and cassava grown in a relay sequence are typically around 500, 500, and 10000 kg ha" in the region respectively.

There would still be a need for fallow periods of over 25 years to restore the harvested Ca and 60 years for K. However, fire-free land preparation based on mulching implies the slow release of nutrients and leads to dramatic yield reductions of nearly 50%, which would not be attractive to farmers. Through the application of moderate amounts of NPK fertilizer, these differences in performance between the two land preparation methods could be partly eliminated, but the K and Ca balance would remain problematic from a sustainability standpoint. The ability of trees to serve as a nutrient pump, scavenging nutrients released over the entire rooting depth of the vegetation and bringing them to the surface, has been known for over 100 years. In the eastern Amazon's secondary forests we found roots down to 6 m. Nearly 30%of the root biomass, which varied between 20 and 30 t" ha", was present in soil layers below 1 m. Moreover, estimated water extraction by the vegetation below a depth of 1 m exceeded 300 mm during the dry season thus providing conditions in which a nutrient pump could be active. However, with subsoil exchangeable K and Ca values below 0.01 and 0.1 cmol(-) kg-" between 150 and 600 cm, respectively, the scavenging of at least K appears unlikely. Unless adequate amounts can be liberated through weathering, these elements will have to be applied.

In contrast to K, which has to be deliberately supplied, the requirement of Ca as a plant nutrient is often inadvertently covered by the application of Cabearing P fertilizers SSP or phosphate rock. Most compound fertilizers lack Ca, thus requiring special measures to assure a positive balance. Mamaril et al. demonstrated in an experiment with an acid Ultisol in the Philippines that annual applications of small amounts of lime (0.75 or 1.5 t ha-") sustained yield levels for six years. Such application rates are considered affordable for the resource-poor farmer.

Modern agriculture

Rice cultivation in the wetland regions of South and South-east Asia has evolved from a traditional practice, with stable yields over millennia, into an intensive form of agriculture within a period of a few decades. Yields appear to have been stable at around 1000±2000 kg ha-", which posed low to moderate demands on the soil for nutrients. Between 1936 and 1952, grain yields in over 3000 fertilizer trials were slightly over 1700 kg ha-" in the absence of N-fertilizer (Yates et al. 1953, cited by De Geus. Sharsabuddhi estimated the associated nutrient removal by grain and straw for a crop of rice in India at 32 kg ha-" of N, 10 kg ha-" of P and 56 kg ha-" of K. Takahashi reported removal by the crop (grain and straw) in Japan of 17 kg of N, 4 kg of P and 22 kg of K for each tonne of rough grain. Similar figures were reported for Taiwan by Chiu with 20 kg of N, 4 kg of P and 20 kg of K for each tonne of rice grain, of which 8 kg of N, 1 kg of P and 16.5 kg of K were in the straw.

Thus, if straw is left in the field, a large share of the nutrients will be returned, particularly K. The long-term productivity of rice paddies was traditionally assured through natural inputs such as biological nitrogen fixation and the rejuvenation of the soils by inundating water and weathering of soil minerals. The stability of the system, sometimes over thousands of years, allows an estimation of these inputs based on the outputs of 15±25 kg of N, 3±5 kg of P and 10±15 kg of K ha-" yr-", depending on yield level and the rate of residue restitution. The same principle of steady state would have held true for the secondary and micronutrients. With increasing opportunities for double or even triple cropping, and with yields of rice moving through the ten tonne barrier, nutrient extraction rates in intensive agriculture have greatly increased.

Von Uexkull (1976) tabulated extraction rates to reach around 109 kg of N, 25 kg of P and 142 kg of K ha-" yr-", with annual double crop yields of approximately 6 t when no fertilizer application or straw restitution took place. Our calculations are more conservative, particularly with regard to K. Still, at such rates of nutrient extraction the assumed yields of grain of 3 t ha-″ season-″ would not be sustainable. However, rice straw in modern rice cultures is largely returned to the fields, which would reduce the removal of N, P and K from the field to 72 kg ha-″ of N, 18 kg ha-″ of P and 21 kg of K ha-″. With recommended fertilizer rates of 100 kg N ha-″, 26 kg P ha-″ and 50 kg K ha-″ on average per season, the nutrient balance is more than restored even if 10 t ha-″.yr-″ of grain were the combined yield. In fact, fertilizer use on cereals has seen a meteoric rise over the past 30 years and is re¯ected directly in cereal production. In the early Nineties, 7 Mt of N (100 kg N ha-″) were applied on around 70 million hectares of irrigated rice of South, East and South-east Asia, with a mean yield of rice of 5 t ha-″. However, with N:P:K ratios in the region of 1:0.15:0.1 actual application rates of P and K are below those recommended, approaching a mere 15 kg P and 10 kg K. Moreover, N fertilizer losses in rice are notoriously high, reaching 30±50% of the applied N, negating possible N gains.

The lesson to be extracted from these calculations is that nutrient budgets in agro-ecosystems are fragile and adapt poorly to the pressures associated with intensification of agriculture. In the West, a concerted effort has been made to find means of assessing the amounts of nutrients needed to supplement those provided by the soil. After four decades of intensive agriculture, we have belatedly recognized that these methods are inadequate, and the approach may need to be changed altogether. The alternative approach involves a closing of the nutrient cycles at the agroecosystem level to the extent possible, and a replenishment of all nutrients that are taken out of the system, in order to conserve the resource base.

Constraints to Fertilizer Adoption

Constraints that may prevent the adoption of fertilizers can be related to a lack of access to markets, unfavourable market prices, as well as to climatic and edaphic uncertainties. In the least developed economies, factors such as lack of money or credit, and unfamiliarity with fertilizer predominate, as was demonstrated in surveys of farmers in Ghana, Togo and Niger. Moreover, farm gate costs of fertilizers in such countries often far exceed those in developed economies, due to excessive marketing costs. In West African countries, these add between 22 and 43% to the total cost of fertilizer, of which transportation takes the lion's share, 39% on average. In less accessible countries such as Zambia and Ethiopia transportation costs are 50% or more of the marketing costs. Short of subsidies there are few short term remedies to overcome the problems associated with market prices and access. Subsidy policies vary enormously by country and product. In 1988}89 subsidies on fertilizers ranged from 6±12% in Togo to 60±67% in neighbouring Ghana. Rapidly changing subsidy policies, often imposed by donors' structural adjustment plans, provide little stability in long-term planning by farmers.

Farming is a business, and as such is interested in efficiency of resource utilization and reasonable returns on investments. As agriculture intensified in Europe and the USA, soil-testing services emerged as a means of optimizing the use of fertilizers, one of the most important cash outlays by the farmer at the time. A host of soil tests were developed to assess the extent to which plant requirements could be met from the soil, which, together with yield targets and nutrient requirements of the specific crop formed the basis for fertilizer recommendations. The considerable investment made in this methodology has not been able to prevent inefficiencies, leading to substantial accumulations of plant nutrients and the Phil. Trans. R. Soc. Lond. B associated pollution in some highly intensified agricultural and horticultural regions of the modern world.

This is due, in part, to the decreasing relative cost of fertilizers for Western farmers, which has led to wasteful application rates. Environmental concerns and a more competitive agriculture are now leading to precision nutrient management. In the tropics, fertilizer still constitutes one of the main costs associated with crop production. Most tropical countries have adopted soil-testing methods from the USA, but few services are available to farmers. Moreover, adequate critical levels have yet to be established for most tropical crops. For those that have been studied in more detail, correlations between these tests and the response to the respective nutrients in the field are poor. In part, this may be due to the importance of SOM and the soil biomass in the maintenance of soil fertility in the tropics. Since the role of SOM diminishes with long term fertilization most soil-testing methods were not designed to capture the important contribution that SOM can make in the course of the season to crops' nutrient requirements. Recently, new efforts are being made to capture these dynamic aspects of soil fertility. The complexity of many cropping systems found in the tropics is further complicating the development of fertilizer recommendations. In short, a major effort is needed to develop better methods of assessing the fertilizer needs for tropical crops and cropping systems. More importantly, methods are needed to evaluate the long-term effects of fertilizer use and the sustainability of fertilizer-based systems, particularly in the more fragile environments, in order to guide farmers better in their quest to meet the growing food demand.

Risk is a problem facing many farmers using fertilizers in the tropics. These risks can be biotic and abiotic in nature. Biotic constraints have led to a dramatic surge in the use of biocides, whereas some abiotic constraints are overcome through irrigation drought), subsoiling liming soil acidity, or drainage. For instance, fertilizer use in the semi-arid tropics can be profitable, particularly if combined with improved cultural practices and High Yielding Varieties. In dry years, however, response to N may not pay for the investment or, in extreme cases can be negative due to impaired grain production. Nitrogen or other nutrients may frequently be more limiting to crop growth in the SAT than water, and may lead to poor water-use efficiency when rainfall is adequate. Moreover, soil nitrate can be left unused in the soil in the absence of rainfall, or be lost through leaching by excessive rains. The complexities of these interactions give rise to highly variable yields and use efficiencies of applied N. The high risk is re‾ected in low fertilizer adoption rates in the SAT regions, covering around 2000 million hectares (Ryan 1974) and supporting more than 900 million people, according to recent information from International Crops Research Institute for the Semi-Arid Tropics. In India, where the efforts to reach the SAT farmer are probably the most intensive, fertilizer consumption increased ten-fold between 1970-1971 and 1985-1986, but still amounts to less than 10%of the Indian N consumption.

In those regions where adequate returns on investment cannot be guaranteed, the farmer's options to increase long-term crop production are rather limited. Bationo & Mokwunye argue convincingly that good organic matter management is the key to soil fertility management. Research results reported by them and those summarized by Pieri show that no less than 15±20 t ha-" of manure are needed to obtain the effect otherwise achieved by chemical fertilizers. Young estimated requirements of crop residues to range from 2 t ha-" in the semi-arid zones to over 8 t ha-" for the humid tropical regions.

With the many alternative needs for organic material such quantities are not generally available. The best one probably could hope for is that organic matter levels be maintained, through a combination of crop residue restitution, fallowing, or green manuring. The positive experience in India with incorporation of legumes in the cropping system was recently reviewed by Lee & Wani. Numerous other constraints can depress the efficiency and profitability of fertilizer use. Soil acidity is one of the most serious problems, affecting an area of 580 million hectares of potentially arable land in the humid tropics. The key nutritional disorders in acid soils are related to toxic manganese and aluminium levels, the associated lack of phosphorus, and the secondary nutrients S, Ca and Mg. The common solution to these problems is liming to pH levels around 6.5, where P availability is judged to be maximized and Al toxicity is eliminated. The primary effect of lime is to reduce the free Al-species, which, as was shown for an acid Ultisol in Malaysia, correlates well with crop yield. Lime or dolomitic lime also serves as a source of Ca and}or Mg. Most commonly, the liming rate is based on the titration curve established for the soil type in question. In the case of Oxisols, Reeve & Sumner recommend basing lime requirements on the exchangeable Al index. Responses to up to 10 t of lime are not uncommon, and residual effects may last several years. Such recommendations are of little use to small farmers that could ill-afford these investments without government support. They were, however, adopted by the Brazilian Government as a condition of sale of Cerrado land, together with substantial investments in P and Zn. Thus, 50 million hectares of land were opened up for agriculture, mostly for mechanized farming on larger farm holdings.

Phosphate application rates needed to satisfy the fixing capacity of acid soils may vary considerably. The low-fixing acid soils of West Africa require as little as 13 kg ha-″ P to support crop growth adequately, whereas the high-fixing acid soils of Latin America will show little crop response with P Phil. Trans. R. Soc. Lond. B (1997) rates below 88 kg ha-″ P, although much higher application rates are common. The cost to the farmer may be prohibitive. One of the attractive options extensively studied in the past decades has been the application of phosphate rock (PR) as a slow-release source of P and Ca for direct application on acid soils.

The topic has been exhaustively reviewed by Khasawneh & Doll (1978) and Hammond et al. (1986). Although some details on the optimum management practices are still being argued, there is little doubt that direct application of PR, many deposits of which are found in the tropics, provides a low cost option to supply P to acid soils. The effectiveness of application not only depends on soil characteristics, but also on the quality of the PR. The reactivity of tropical PRs varies widely, leading to differences in the availability of P from these sources.

If low P availability is primarily related to low native P levels in soil, P additions are unavoidable if soil productivity is to be restored. Whether this P originates from neighbouring pastures and is added as manure, or from subsoil P reserves pumped to the surface through fallow vegetation, or from chemical fertilizers, is up to the farmer. In general, he will be basing his choice on land and resource availability considerations. In high fixing soils, a number of alternatives are being studied. One of these options is to look for crops or crop varieties that have a greater tolerance for low soil P. Many plant species have developed mechanisms to help overcome P constraints by reducing the distance to the P source through increased root growth, improved acid tolerance, an increased exudation of P-solving acids or chelates or with the help of omnipresent mycorrhiza.

The Need for Fertilizers and Recycling

Fertilizer supplies are assured in the coming century. Nitrogen is involved in a cycle between the atmosphere and the biosphere with rates of fixation by electrical discharges, and biological and industrial processes of 250 Mt yr-". At this rate the atmosphere could supply N for about 20 million years but would sooner run out of O. The fixed N is largely returned by denitrification, with little net accrual globally. As long as energy is available to transform it to the ammoniacal form, the nitrogen supply is assured. Phosphate reserve estimates vary from 3.4 to 51 Gt of P, dependent on what is considered economically feasible. Fertilizer consumption in 1990 amounted to 16 Mt yr-"of P. Even with the lowest estimate of 3.4 Gt of P by the Global 2000 model, P reserves would represent a supply for 90±130 years. However, considering the estimated 23 Mt yr-" of P that are irretrievably lost to the oceans, P use may have to be increased to compensate for this waste. Somewhere between 29 and 93 Gt of K reserves are documented, and others are known to exist that have yet to be explored. At the current rate of production of around 21 Mt yr-" of K, these reserves will last another millennium.

Trade in fertilizers and crop and livestock commodities is leading to a net transfer of nutrients from producing continents to the consuming regions. The net movement of P amounts to a transfer from North and Central America and North Africa to Asia and Europe. The resulting accumulations in P, depicted in figure 2, are translated into accrual rates of around 30 kg P ha-", causing serious problems in some regions with highly intensified agriculture. The P accrual rates for Africa and Latin America are likely to be insufficient to compensate for losses due to erosion and accumulations in city waste, and are consistent with the warnings of serious nutrient mining in Africa.

Nearly half the current population (2.6 billion) are city dwellers, two-thirds of them inhabit the developing world. The population growth in the coming ten years (0.7 billion) will almost entirely end up in cities. The rural population will be increasingly in¯uenced by urban centres, as it will be called upon to produce food for its population. On the other hand, the recent migrants, constituting around 40% of the growth in urban populations, increasingly rely on urban agriculture to cover part of their food needs. With current urban expansion rates, nutrients in harvested products are increasingly lost from the rural environment as a whole.

Closing the nutrient cycle at a community level in rural areas may be tedious: on an inter-regional level it is associated with considerable costs of collection, detoxification and transportation to the farms. Yet, at the rate at which some of the non-renewable resources such as P and K are being exploited, recycling of these nutrients will soon be required. Here indeed, political foresight is needed to translate our awareness into action programmes. Very few examples exist today of Phil. Trans. R. Soc. Lond. B (1997) 982 P. L. G. Vlek and others Nutrient resources regions that purposely set out to close the disrupted nutrient cycle. In fact, the increasing problems in disposing of household garbage and sewage are causing many advanced communities to reassess their energy and material ¯ows. For a middle-sized urban community in Switzerland, Baccini & Bader estimate that of the 1000 kg of consumables entering a private household per person per year, approximately 600 kg end up in sewage and 50 kg as compostable materials. Around 80% of the P ¯owing through the urban household enters as food. Of the 5 kg of P and 18 kg of N that enter the aboveground parts of the crops per person per year to produce food, about 1 kg of P and 8 kg of N actually leave the farm and are eventually discarded in sewage.

Environmental awareness is putting pressure on farmers to shift their strategy towards soil fertility maintenance based on natural resource conservation, biological nitrogen fixation, and input efficiency. The continuation or adoption of these resource conservation techniques requires awareness by the farmer of the long-term consequences of soil mining. In contrast to soil erosion, the process of soil mining is not obvious and is difficult to discern, even though the ultimate consequences are not. Under the pressures of meeting the food demands of a region, farmers are often encouraged to adopt fertilizer practices. Often, the success of these chemicals is tempting farmers to abandon sound agronomic practices, such as mixed cropping. In China alone, millions of hectares of A.olla-based rice paddies have been turned into ureabased monocultures. As long as the products remain within the community, the nutrient cycle can be restored if the political will exists and the necessary infrastructure and incentives are provided.

The strategy of closing the nutrient cycle at the farm level by using fallow fields, returning residues, and maintaining the biologically fixing organisms, is often referred to as integrated soil fertility management. Using the latest knowledge regarding cultural practices, cropping systems and nutrient cycles, it aims to optimize and stabilize agricultural production within a given ecological and socio-economic environment. Nutrient depletion, as well as accumulation, is avoided but imbalances are corrected. Integrated soil fertility management does not preclude the use of fertilizers, but weighs their use against the alternatives in terms of direct and long-term environmental costs in meeting the demand for food and fibre. The resulting strategies may differ considerably for similar ecosystems due to varying infrastructure, population or policy settings, resulting in different market conditions. Therefore, it is difficult to provide a blueprint for nutrient management in defined environments without considering these externalities. The concept is equally applicable to marginal and favourable environments, irrespective of their current soil nutrient status. Principles of mixed cropping, alley cropping, residue conservation or fallowing are, however, slow to find their way back into modern agriculture, and where these practices are still existent they are in fact disappearing, e.g. the A.olla-based rice culture in China. The resulting soil degradation spells hunger for future generations. As we enter a new millennium, we will have to come to terms with these different short- and long-term expectations from our natural resource base.

17

Big Farms, Small Farms: Strategies in Sustainable Agriculture

Given the continuing trend towards larger farms – 2% of farms now produce 35% of the food in Canada this paper proposes that strategies for sustainable agriculture must include both small and large farms. Small farms may meet the non-economic criteria for sustainability but they have not been able to remain economically viable in the modern context; with substantial and increasing divergence between the different sizes of farms, there needs to be differentiated treatment of the two principle types of agricultural operations.

Paying for Sustainability

Canadian agricultural policy and programs need to integrate ecological parameters into income support measures similar to the revised Common Agricultural Policy for the European Union. These also need to go further than just eco-compliance and provide income assistance through environmental enhancement programs where of all of society benefit from the results such as protecting wetlands. Other suggested measures for supporting sustainability are:

- A consumer levy on food to provide farmers with a stabilized and equitable income to enable greater adoption rates for sustainable practices.
- Greater exploitation of biomass for energy, both for off-farm fuel products ethanol, biodiesel) and onfarm energy substitution electricity from manure.

Safe and Nutritious Food

Although there is considerable effort being made with regard to food safety regulations and systems there are some larger questions which require strategic approaches in terms of food safety and nutrition.

- Trust The creation of an independent food authority along the lines of a commissioner's office to provide an arm's length review of the scientific and regulatory issues related to food safety would be a big step towards re-building consumer trust.
- Transparency The approval process for agri-food technologies is not as transparent as it could be and should be addressed through improved processes that support peer review and independent verification of research findings.

  Understanding there is substantial confusion surrounding food issues in the public domain, and there is a need for a national centre with a specific focus on communications and education related to issues in the agri-food sector.
- Traceability the capacity to track food back to its point of origin risks undermining one of the important tenants of sustainability - small farms - through burdensome regulations and paperwork. Elements of practicality are required in these systems which respond to farm size.
- Nutrition utilization of modern information technology could be better applied to provide consumers with

detailed nutritional information.

- MPI minimal process interference could become an indicator of sustainability by showing just how far evolved a particular food product is from its natural state, including the use of crop protection materials, processing changes and additions, and packaging and distribution.
- Future foods The 'disassembly' of whole foods into constituent parts is now beginning to move forward into the molecular realm. Such capacity has huge implications for questions of sustainability and requires discussion and debate before the products appear on supermarket shelves.

Vibrant Rural Communities

There is an exodus from Canada's rural communities, in particular farming ones. Rather than looking at strategies to only increase the number of small farms, this paper proposes approaches that look at ways in which agriculture can make a contribution to the vibrancy of rural communities, big farm or small.

- Owner operator local ownership of farms, regardless of farm structure, should be encouraged to ensure greater socio-economic commitment to the local community by larger farms.
- Value Added the presence of local post-production processing and or distribution facilities creates employment and economic development opportunities, and should be encouraged.
- Strategic Alliances – the notion of exchange and or co-operation between farmers in order to provide greater critical mass in terms of production and processing capacity need to be formalized and expanded in order to maintain farm numbers while providing benefits from economies of scale.

- Farm succession – intergenerational transfers must be better facilitated if there is going to be a next generation of farmers in Canada.
- Fiscal – both federal and provincial governments have progressively removed many of the fiscal incentives that made the 'cash poor, paper rich' nature of farming viable. Rejuvenated fiscal strategies would be welcome support for encouraging young farmers.
- Non-farming farmers new programs are needed to facilitate partial farm ownership or share cropping as further incentive for re-engagement of non-farmers in agriculture and, therefore, rural communities.
- Immigration Few immigrants choose to settle in rural communities. Some possibilities to encourage immigration into rural communities are more flexible provisions for immigrant professionals to be able to work in rural areas, allowances for overseas seasonal workers to become landed immigrants, and development of social structures to assist new arrivals, such as community-owned cooperative housing, to settle in rural areas.

Conservation of Resources and Environment

Much attention has been paid to the environmental impact of agriculture in the last 20 years, and, as a consequence, a variety of policies, programs, and regulations have been developed such as water protection policies, environmental farm plans and nutrient management plans. Most have targeted containment pollution reduction or focused on management practices. The five major aspects in this regard and their targeted results are:

- Livestock facilities All facilities should be leakage free with tolerable but minimal odour and dust.
- Nutrient management Application of nutrients to meet crop needs while maintaining optimal crop yields and

soil fertility, and to minimize the risk of nutrient run-off and leaching.

- Soil erosion - Soil erosion is reduced to a level where soil productivity can be maintained for the foreseeable future, and its impact on water quality in permanent watercourses does not prevent the water from meeting current standards for maximal usage.

- Energy efficiency - The farm should generate true carbon credits, and the energy efficiencies achieved are at least such that if the harvested biomass from a farm was to be converted into ethanol, the amount of energy in the ethanol would exceed the energy expenditure used for the production, transport and treatment of the raw biomass.

- Biodiversity - Wetlands, highly sensitive lands, forested lands that are inadequate for agriculture should be protected, and watercourses should be targeted as corridors for both wildlife shelter and restored as routes for animal migration

Other strategic elements that should be considered in minimizing environmental risks and conserving natural resources:

- Watershed management - management by watershed objectives enables the participation of all interested stakeholders, the establishment of benchmarks and the measurement of site-specific improvements.

- Windbreaks - soil erosion is a major pathway by which nutrients and other pollutants reach watercourses.

Further improvement can be achieved through the establishment of windbreaks which have the added benefit of diversifying habitat.

- Energy higher fossil fuel prices present potential opportunities for farmers to enhance local production by displacing imported food that becomes more expensive to transport, and the generation of energy from biomass sources for on-farm use and sales to energy providers.

Research and Extension

Progression in agricultural sustainability requires systems information knowledge rather than just new applied technologies, and this aspect is threatened by the decline and/or transformation of the research and extension network which warrants new approaches.

- Research levy – A levy on commodities will be necessary to inject new funds into research and extension on sustainable agricultural practices.
- Producer-operated extension structures – New structures are required to ensure that extension services are available to all farmers on an unconditional basis.
- Information technologies – Some farms are still on party lines and cannot use a fax; there needs to be the creation of programs and provisions that allow the comprehensive uptake of advances in information technologies in rural areas.

Incentives, Regulations and Indicators

The imposition of a regulatory framework regarding sustainable agriculture is likely to further accelerate the trend towards bigger farms, for which there needs to be strategic responses.

- Variable regulations – Agri-environmental regulations need to be modulated to reflect the particular situation of individual farms and support variable applicability (on a farm-by-farm basis.)
- More management – environmental management aspects have to be integrated in conjunction with the regulatory framework. The movement toward individual environmental farm plans is an example of

one such strategy.

- Incentives – While regulations set the framework, incentives are the positive reinforcement, and the identification of opportunities whereby farmers can be compensated for providing a service would greatly assist in the incorporation of sustainable practices.
- Indicators – A considerable amount of work has already been done on identifying what the indicators should be, the next step needs to be to work out what should be benchmarked, how is that to be carried out, and what is the level of change to be achieved?

The purpose of this paper, as defined by the Agricultural Institute of Canada is to inform the discussion and debate on the issue of sustaining agriculture in Canada. This has been carried out through a comprehensive review of scientific research and credible literature, and includes background information on sustainable agriculture and an exploration of the various issues pertaining to sustainability. This has been carried out within the definition of sustainable agriculture as determined by AIC (for the purposes of this discussion paper):

The application of husbandry experience and scientific knowledge of natural processes to create agriculture and agri-food systems that are economically viable and meet society's need for safe and nutritious food and vibrant rural communities, while conserving or enhancing natural resources and the environment.

This definition is *grosso mondo,* consistent with most descriptions of sustainable agriculture given that it addresses the major elements that have an impact in this area – the environmental, social and economic aspects that inter-relate with agri-food activities. The reference to husbandry experience and scientific knowledge is, of course, particular to AIC's membership being that they are directly involved with food production, and the organization's role in providing information on science-based solutions regarding environmental sustainability, food safety and food sufficiency.

Background

Despite the fact that the basics of farming function pretty much the same as they have since humans began to collect seeds from harvest to re-plant the following year, and to domesticate animals for the purposes of planned food production, agriculture has changed significantly in the way it functions over the last 100 years. Agriculture has changed due to the introduction of the combustion engine and electricity for power, the advent of synthetic fertilizers and crop protection materials, and the non-stop arrival of new technologies. From hydraulics to artificial insemination to genetically engineered crops, changes have been significant. The corn stalk still grows upright in the field, but nothing about the way it grows and how it is harvested and processed has been left untouched by the 'green revolution'. Agriculture, previously considered more of a socio-cultural component of human society, has rapidly developed, along with the processing of food, to become commoditized, industrialized and globalized within the last 50 years. In developed nations, and increasingly in developing nations such as Brazil which is now a major commodity exporter, agriculture has become a significant part of the modern economy; in Canada in 2002, the bio-food sector contributed $113 billion, or 12% of GDP and over half of the sector's vitality depends on exports outside the region of production (interprovincial and international)1; in 2004, agri-food exports amounted to $24 billion, shipments growing at a rate of more than 10% annually.2 The changes have brought considerable increases in productivity for a hungry world, and greatly minimized the risks that farmers have to face in bringing in a crop.

Like all industrialized sectors, the benefits have also produced negative impacts, in particular the 'footprint' that farming has left on the ecology that provides the basic components to produce food: soil degradation, contaminated and depleted water sources, poor air quality and reduced biodiversity. The human ecology has also been impacted with a tremendous drop in farm numbers, an on-going exodus from rural areas and poor economic and working conditions for those engaged and employed in the sector. The capacity of humancreated technologies and processes has extracted from nature many benefits, but at the same time has become overpowering, particularly in the shadow of unrelenting population growth. Mother Earth may have been able to absorb uncontrolled expansion and exploitation if there were just a billion people, but as world population reached and passed three and four and five billions of people, the evidence became clear: the human presence on earth, unless it changed, was becoming unsustainable.

Thus the emergence of the term 'sustainable development', and, as applied to farming, sustainable agriculture. In essence, how can human society continue to feed itself without destroying the environment, contaminating the food that comes from the natural landscape, and rendering the surrounding communities uninhabitable? "If civilization is to survive, it must live on the interest, not the capital of nature. Ecological markers suggest that in the early 1960s, humans were using about 70 per cent of nature's yearly output; by the early 1980s, we'd reached 100 per cent; and in 1999, we were at 125 per cent. Such numbers may be imprecise, but their trend is clear – they mark the road to bankruptcy."

The response to such predictions has been a rapid evolution of thinking and planning related to agricultural production, moving from awareness of the need for change into research, education, policy development, strategies for implementation and ultimately, action itself. Whole movements have emerged around issues of sustainability in human affairs – sustainable energy, sustainable transportation, even sustainable tourism.

Only agriculture carries with it a double burden: we can use less energy for heating by insulating our homes better, we can improve air quality by using mass transit systems more effectively, we can reduce the evergrowing ecological footprint of tourism by staying at home more often. But we still have to eat everyday, and make sure that there is enough food for the additional 6 billion people that are expected to fill this planet in the next century. Agriculture is different as it faces the double challenge of continuing to expand production while trying to maintain its sustainability.

What is Agricultural Sustainability

Different definitions of sustainability and there are many – generally revolve around the core elements described at the beginning of this paper: economic viability, safe food, vibrant rural communities and environmental conservation. Sustainability is, however, in the eye of the beholder, and very much related to not just the choice of words used in the description but also their interpretation. One definition maintains that to "be sustainable, human activity, as well as the means to carry it out, must be capable of being continued indefinitely". Other common descriptions often utilized are "long-term", "foreseeable future" and, in the case of the definition used in this paper, there is no reference to timeline at all.

But rather than getting stuck on the meaning of "healthy" versus "safe and nutritious", the examination of sustainability is better viewed in terms of goals, objectives and indicators – what are we aiming for, how will this be achieved and, most importantly, how will we know we've arrived (or more appropriate to the context of sustainability, how far along the journey have we traveled.) The goals and objectives have been set, and much work has been done on indicators.4 The real challenge is implementation, potential strategies for action which are presented later in this paper.

Exploration of Issues and Conflicts in Sustainability

Following is a brief description of the key issues (adapted in part from Agriculture and Agri-Food Canada, Sustainable Development Strategy and the University of California)6 and dichotomies related to sustainability in agriculture.

Water Quality and Use *Nutrients*

Nutrients are applied to crops in the form of chemical

fertilizers or manure. Used sustainably, these inputs help maintain soil health and increase productivity and economic returns. However, applied in excess or under the wrong conditions, they may contribute to the pollution of surface water and groundwater, negatively affect yields, and waste farm resources. Some excess nutrients, such as nitrates, can pose a human health risk when concentration levels in drinking water exceed guidelines.

Pathogens

Pathogens are disease-causing agents, such as bacteria or viruses. Where pathogen concentrations from agricultural outputs such as manure run-off into water systems exceed drinking water guidelines for surface water or groundwater, negative effects on human health may result.

Pesticides

Controlling pests and diseases is fundamental to the production of safe, high-quality, and abundant agricultural products for Canadians. Pesticide residues can make their way into water systems, where they may pose a threat to human health and local ecosystems.

Water Conservation

The sustainable use of water requires that withdrawal rates from water sources not exceed recharge rates or compromise other water uses. On a national level, agriculture uses about nine per cent of the water withdrawn in Canada, mainly to grow crops, water livestock, clean farm buildings and equipment, and meet domestic needs. Although agriculture returns less than 30 percent of the water it uses to its source, a much higher percentage is returned indirectly to the environment.

Particulate Emissions

Farms emit particulate matter as primary particles (most commonly dust from soil erosion and cultivation, and smoke from burning crop residue) and secondary particles (formed in the air from gases emitted by agriculture, such as ammonia). Exposure to particulate matter may have adverse effects on ecosystems and human health.

Odours

Farm odours can cause significant conflict between farmers and neighbouring communities. In some areas such conflicts have given rise to municipal action to control the siting of intensive livestock operations.

Greenhouse Gas Emissions

About 10 per cent of Canada's human-produced greenhouse gas emissions come from agricultural production, excluding the use of fossil fuels or the emissions from fertilizer production. The main greenhouse gases emitted by agricultural activities are nitrous oxide, from fertilizer and animal manure, and methane, from cattle and livestock manure. Carbon dioxide is also emitted from soils and energy combustion. However, agriculture also has the ability to remove carbon dioxide from the atmosphere through cultivation practices which reduce disturbance to soil and enhance the build-up of organic carbon in the soils. Greenhouse gas emissions contribute to climate change.

Soil Erosion

Soil erosion is the redistribution of soil in the landscape by agents such as wind, water, and tillage. The effects of soil erosion on crop quality and yields can be substantial. Erosion may also negatively affect offfarm air and water quality, as well as wildlife habitat.

Soil Organic Matter

Loss of soil organic matter leads to the depletion of soil organic carbon. This results in the breakdown of soil structure, greater vulnerability of the soil to erosion, and reduced fertility. These factors lead to reductions in yield and sustainability of the soil resource. Increased decomposition of soil organic matter contributes to rising levels of atmospheric carbon dioxide, a greenhouse gas implicated in climate change.

Intensive Operations

The consolidation of farming units has resulted in the growth of intensive livestock operations which can house thousands of animal units in one location. This has resulted in increases in 'nuisance' activities such as noise, dust and odours, as well as concerns related to water contamination from manure storage and spreading. The emergence of ILOs has lead to much heavier regulation of farming activities and the development of regulatory and management tools such as environmental farm and nutrient management plans.

Feed Consumption

Modern livestock production depends heavily on the consumption of high energy grains and protein oilseeds. There are concerns that this is an inefficient way of producing food calories, and that direct consumption of grains by humans would help alleviate food shortages in other parts of the world and promote a healthier diet based on less meat consumption. Livestock producers maintain that much of the feed used for livestock production is not as suitable for human consumption and modern genetics have made livestock into much more efficient converters of feed grains in meat protein.

Animal Welfare

Many of the intensively raised livestock are confined in housing that severely limits their space and ability to move around, as well as access to the outside. This has raised ethical questions about the treatment of animals even within their short lifespan, and revisions to livestock housing and welfare codes have been on-going.

Fossil Fuels for Food

Modern agriculture has become a significant consumer of fossil fuel based inputs, from synthetic fertilizers to pesticides. Some estimates peg the caloric ratio of energy consumption to food produced at more than eight to one, a rate that is unsustainable in the long term and contributing to higher food costs as energy prices rise. Minimum tillage, low-input and organic farming methods are increasing in use as ways to address the question of energy dependence.

Equipment

Agricultural production operations run on diesel fuel and electricity, with relative increases as mechanization and production intensity also increase. Farms are experimenting with bio-fuels and electricity generation from manure and other renewable sources (wind, solar.)

Habitat Availability

Loss and alteration of habitat are the leading causes of depletion of the earth's wildlife species, and biodiversity. Conversion of natural land to agriculture has contributed to declining wildlife habitat. However, agriculture offers better habitat than many other land uses by humans, such as urban development.

Species at Risk

The protection of threatened and endangered species is a priority issue both within Canada and internationally. As of May 2000, the Committee on the Status of Endangered Wildlife in Canada determined that 12 Canadian species are extinct and an additional 341 species are at risk. These numbers do not reflect the status of the many invertebrates, micro-organisms, and lower plants that have not yet been evaluated. Many of these species are important agents in the regulation of the ecological processes that underpin sustainable agriculture.

Impact of Wildlife

Wildlife on farmland offer advantages, such as pollination, predation of crop and livestock pests, aesthetic appeal, hunting, and fishing. They also pose some disadvantages, such as reduced crop yield, livestock kills, and damage to buildings.

Forces of Nature

Extreme natural events such as drought, hail, and insect population explosions can have a significant impact on farmers' income. For example, back-to-back droughts on the Prairies in 2001 and 2002 slowed production growth for some crops with value-added potential and created uncertainty for potential investors in processing plants. Droughts and flooding have driven home the importance of sustainable farming practices and income stabilization programs.

Politics of International Trade

Protectionist agriculture policies in other countries, such as trade-distorting domestic support and export subsidies, remain an impediment to expanding world agricultural and agri-food trade. For example, the US Farm Bill and European Union agricultural policies stimulate production and put downward pressure on commodity prices, affecting the competitiveness of Canadian exports in these markets.

Variations in Markets

Markets are not immune to price swings. Producers must cope with changes in commodity prices and market preferences, which are often difficult to predict.

Food Safety

Food safety is a basic requirement for a modern food system. Surveys show that food safety is a key consideration for Canadians who are demanding greater assurances about the food they eat. Recent highprofile incidents involving Bovine Spongiform Ecephalopathy in Europe and Canada, dioxin contamination in Europe, and *E. coli* 0157:H7 in hamburger and unpasteurized juice in North America underline the importance of food safety. Such incidents have notable economic and social consequences, causing significant monetary loss for the sector, and, in some cases posing serious health risks.

Rapidly Evolving Consumer Preferences

Greater public concern about food safety issues is raising

awareness in the sector of the need to adopt common industry standards at the farm and processor levels. As well, consumer interest in how agricultural products are produced, including potential environmental impacts such as pesticides, antibiotics and biotechnology, is growing. This interest is creating new market opportunities for agricultural products produced in environmentally friendly ways, such as organic and reduced-pesticide production.

Threat of Exotic Pests and Fast-moving Diseases

Outbreaks of diseases or pathogens within the food production and processing chain were once isolated in small areas. Today's intensive farming and the greater movement of goods and people have made such threats much more difficult to contain. As a result, outbreaks—whether arising from natural causes or bioterrorism— can spread throughout a country and around the world in a remarkably short time.

Fewer But Larger Farms

Canadians who make up the agriculture and agri-food sector reside mainly in Canada's rural communities. Although, over time, there has been a trend towards significantly larger farms, 98 per cent of all farms are still family-owned and-operated.

Demographics

According to the 2001 Census, the job of running the farm in Canada is increasingly falling to fewer and older farmers. Farm operators also have a median age much higher than the comparable labour force population of self-employed workers. Although reductions in the total number of farmers may reflect increased productivity in the sector, a lack of younger workers entering the field may cause labour shortages in the future.

Employment

Many rural communities have seen their populations falter as employment opportunities decline. This also has an impact on social infrastructure and the capacity of rural communities to remain viable.

Dichotomies

Given the context of modern civilization, sustainability is not an easy concept to tackle at the best of times. It evokes notions of greater responsibility for the world which we inhabit, more discipline in how we exploit its resources and the exercise of better judgment in how we apply the distinctive characteristic of *homo sapiens* the acquisition and use of knowledge. Sustainability with regards to agriculture is even more complex because of its cultural connections to food, the socio-political dynamic of rural decline and the double-duty of feeding the world while conserving the environment. Mass tourism is a relatively new human activity that is stamping its footprint across the world, but there are some pretty straightforward remedies that are impeded not by a lack of viable options but mostly by the tourists overwhelming desire to have a good time come what may. Agriculture doesn't have the same margin of maneuver.

Sustainable agriculture, aside from dealing with the basic approaches of sustainability along the lines of 'reduce, re-use, recycle', also has to resolve a number of dichotomies fundamental to any approach that might be taken to achieve greater levels of sustainability. Left unsettled, these conflicts will, at best, be a hindrance to any substantial progress in this regard, and, at worst, mire the sector in a never-ending debate. It is instructive to note that in 2004 the New Zealand Parliamentary Commissioner for the Environment published a large study on intensive farming and the environment. In early 2005, follow-up workshops with regional agricultural communities were conducted and the evaluations from over 500 participants clearly displayed the divide when it comes to sustainability in agriculture: just over one half agreed that farming was mostly sustainable but that some issues needed to be addressed, and just under one half agreed that farming is mostly unsustainable and change is required at all levels.

Following is a brief description of the important dichotomies related to sustainability in Canadian agriculture. Many of the points raised are touched upon in more detail in other sections of the paper.

Science and Technology

Science and technology have quite clearly helped get us into this mess who knew that those very effective and efficient pellets of fertilizer would also kill fish when leached out of the soil and some believe that science and technology will get us out of it. Amongst several issues in this regard, biotechnology is prominent. Proponents assert that genetically engineered crops and livestock can increase productivity while reducing the need for inputs, thus making agricultural production more sustainable. Opponents contend that biotechnology goes beyond the bounds of acceptable genetic improvement through 'natural' methods of breeding, as well as posing unacceptable risks to the environment and human health and food safety. There are also issues of control (patents and technology agreements), as well as corporate concentration. Half the farming world has readily embraced this new technology, while the other half is battling hard to keep it out; humans have rarely said "no" to technology before, and on what basis do we decide one way or the other, if at all?

Risk/benefit Versus the Precautionary Principle

The foundation of all applications of scientific knowledge is the risk/benefit analysis: what are the risks and to what extent, and what are the benefits and do they outweigh the risks? If the risks are minimal and manageable, and the benefits are substantial and demonstrable, science says that the product or process is safe and useable. The precautionary principle, an outcome of the debates around sustainability, changes the emphasis on the question: if the risks are unknown or unquantifiable, then even if there are benefits, caution should be applied until the risks are known or have been quantified.8 The apparent absence of risk gives the green light under the risk/benefit scenario; the inability to determine risk (as one would determine benefits) and therefore definitively pronounce there is none gives the red light under the precautionary principle. The applied use of molecular technologies, potentially very beneficial to agriculture, may come to a stop unless this difference of assessment is remedied.

Safe Versus Unsafe

Probably the most complex issue within the discussion of sustainability is whether food, as produced in the modern context, is safe or not. Along the lines of biotechnology, there are two camps each claiming that science is on their side, with consumers sitting in the middle saddled with a "once burned, twice shy kind of caution". Are there pesticide and antibiotic residues in food; is it safe to eat foods containing genetically-engineered materials, and what is a safe level anyway? There is a huge volume of data that suggests food is safe as produced using modern practices and technology, and yet there are claims that this is not so. Many of these come from specific instances of environmental contamination, for example a pesticide spill, and from invocation of the precautionary principle - bacteria exposed to antibiotics could become resistant, therefore antibiotics should not be used in food production. Even though systems have been instituted to ensure food safety, there are still many questions to be debated related to the parameters of these systems what is safe in the first place?

Animal Versus Vegetable

Livestock have been an integral part of farming since the beginning of human civilization, and their capacity to consume plant matter otherwise inedible for humans and transform the material into highly nutritious food and fiber could arguably be claimed to be one of the key factors in the establishment of modern civilization. The place of livestock on the pedestal of human society is no more, especially in the developed world where the easy adaptability to intensive production methods has begun to result in livestock being treated as a scourge rather than a resource. Surpluses of manure, odours and consumption of high-energy grains have earned the sector a bad name. On the other hand, manure from livestock is a very valuable fertilizing resource, and meat production can provide better levels of nutrition for the malnourished. In a sector that has become very intensified, what are the factors of sustainability in livestock production?

Intensive Versus Extensive

Until the modern era, much of agriculture was extensive, and until the advent of modern technologies all civilizations that engaged in intensive production without regard to basic agronomic principles failed not only in producing food but also contributed to the collapse of the civilizations themselves.9 Today, with virtually all the available agricultural land already under cultivation, and any remaining areas of the planet likely to be fragile or marginal, there are few options other than to intensify production in order to produce yet more food; intensification can lead to environmental problems, such as salinity from irrigation, which runs counter to the tenets of sustainability. Extensive production alone cannot meet the growing food requirements of the human population and would demand more farm land than there is available. When and where is it appropriate to follow one production path or the other?

Economics Versus Culture

Even in this time of fast food outlets, eating food is an essential element of human culture. Loaded with tradition and blessed with emotion, the culture of food is frequently raised as an element of sustainability. Conversely, the human population has not only embraced but actively sought a secure and cheap source of foodstuffs, driving the commoditization and commercialization of food. Food production is now an integral part of the global economy with freight car loads of grain being treated in the same manner as containers full of widgets. Is modern, commoditized agri-food production now a part of our culture as well?

One Planet Versus Many Worlds

The evolution of human society is one of concentration and

consolidation: single cities bigger than entire nations, nation-blocks occupying large segments of continents (EU), regions becoming one global economy. The world is headed economically and structurally in one direction, sustainability calls for more emphasis on local production. Can these two seemingly opposite forces co-exist within the parameters of sustainability?

Rural Versus Urban

The farming population, once prevalent in rural areas, has diminished to the extent that even in regions where agriculture is predominant, farmers and their families average less than 15% of the rural population, often well below 10%.11 The urban population knows less and less about how food is produced, and very often seems to care little beyond the cost/quality assessment that every item in the grocery receives when being considered for purchase: what am I getting and how much will it cost? Urban expansion is continually eating up prime farm land that surrounds cities and, once the urban perimeter has become established, town folk want to know nothing about the nuisances of farming practices.

Structural Evolution of Farming in Canada

Many of the issues related to sustainable agriculture have been attributed, in part, to the intensification of agriculture exhibited through the increasing use of technology, higher rates of capitalization and consolidation of farming units. In effect, farms have become bigger, investing more in capital expenditures and adopting technology on a continuous – some would even argue – on an addictive basis. This structural evolution is mostly characterized throughout the reviewed literature on sustainable agriculture as 'big is bad, small is beautiful' an assessment reached mostly on the basis that larger farms employing intensive production practices have been chiefly responsible for the consequences described in the introduction (environmental degradation, etc.). Invariably, proponents of sustainability portray the benefits of small farms as the best way to attain increased levels of sustainability in agriculture. There is some truth to this description, but not necessarily the whole truth. The increasing size of farms and the adoption of modern chemical and other technologies have resulted in environmental problems and social dislocations. Small farms respond to many of the criteria elaborated as necessary to achieve sustainability, while the legacy of larger farm units often makes it difficult to see them in the same light. Smaller-sized, family farms (defined in this paper using the threshold of less than $100,000 in gross sales) are touted as the route to sustainability and, if only government policies, markets and regulations were more favorable, these farms would be viable.

The difficulty of this paradigm, however, is that the reality is very much different. Farming in Canada is headed the other way as a greater percentage of the remaining farms are increasing in size because under current economic parameters, it's the only way to stay in business. If the trend continues – and the certain impact in this regard of BSE on farm exits has not yet been registered in the databases – then there will be at a minimum 10% fewer farmers every five years, meaning that in twenty years there will be 35% fewer farmers than today. In addition, given that 30% of today's farmers are producing 70% of the food16, and 2% are producing 35% , a much higher proportion of the remaining farmers in twenty years are going to be classified as *large* farms defined in this paper using the threshold of at least $500,000 in gross sales.

While large farms are usually portrayed as pushing small farms out, it is also a case of picking up the pieces after farmers operating smaller units decide to quit. The reasons are quite clear small farmers grow tired of hard, physical labour that pays so little that they must hold at least a part-time job off the farm in order to earn a decent salary. The benefits of operating a small family farm are quite clearly related to family heritage, lifestyle and other social factors, but outside of particular niche markets, they are not economical in the current context.

And this is not a new trend. Dave McIntosh, in "When the work's all done this fall the settling of the land"19, extracted from the National Archives of Canada a treasure trove of anecdotes, letters, and memoirs relating to the early rural development of Canada. On numerous occasions he records instances where the farmers were eager to get away from the back-breaking labour of farming and move onto greener pastures, or encouraged family members to work as domestic or manufacturing labour for the cash wages. The initial increase in the number of farmers in Canada did not come so much from the off-spring of farmers becoming farmers (French-speaking Quebec being an exception) but from a continual stream of non-farming immigrants seeking a better life; once the mass emigrations to rural Canada ceased in the early part of the 20th Century, so the decline in farm numbers begins. Today, in 21st Century rural Canada, there are very few people lining up to become farmers, and most of those who could inherit a farm are choosing not to do so as is evident from the continuing exit rate from the farm sector. Small may be beautiful, but not at the going price.

Rather than speak of only small farms, this paper proposes that strategies for sustainable agriculture in Canada include both small and large farms. This is a practical approach derived from the following assessment:

- Small farmers are exiting the sector at an increasing rate each census period, a trend that will not likely subside given the current income situation for Canadian farmers21 and the aging farm population without comparable numbers indicating a willingness and capacity to take over as the next generation;
- Continuing reductions in federal and provincial government programs and services that would be essential to maintaining smaller farms (i.e. extension), as well as policies that actually encourage small farmers to do something else – politely referred to as "renewal" in the terminology of Agriculture & Agri-Food

Canada's "Sustainable Development Strategy."

- Macro-economic trends that point towards continued decreases in farm gate prices23, continued increases in productivity through applications of new technologies and the continued opening of world markets and global trade in food commodities all parameters that mitigate against the maintenance of smaller farms.

Regardless of what an individual believes should be changed at the World Trade Organization, in the structure and operations of transnational corporations, and about the introduction of new technologies such as genetically engineered organisms, these are factors already in play and likely to be so at least in the medium term (15-20 years). Any changes and there will be some are more likely to come about through political action, but the predictability and extent of that change (related to impacts on sustainability) are anybody's guess. In the meantime, developing and implementing strategies leading towards greater sustainability through the 'application of husbandry experience and scientific knowledge of natural processes' for all components of Canadian agriculture seems to be a far more pragmatic and productive approach.

Again, in all the reviewed literature, a singular treatment was accorded to the subject of agricultural sustainability - one size of analysis and suggested action fits all types of farms. Given that there are substantial and increasing differences between the different sizes of farms, there needs to be differentiated treatment of the two principle types of farms that, regardless of the subdivisions of categorization, are beginning to dominate the farming landscape: "operators who run large-scale businesses and operators who treat farming as a secondary income".

This treatment need not be entirely exclusive as the sustainability of each of these classes of farms is tied in some respects to the development of the other. Small farms need large farms, and vice-versa:

- Large farms will be able to provide custom operations that small farms can no longer afford to maintain or which must comply to more demanding levels of regulation, as well as serving as local points of trade, exchange and service for supplies, commodities and expertise that might otherwise not exist or be as readily available;
- Small farms will provide large farms with seasonal and experienced labour that is very difficult to find through regular employment channels, as well as contributing to the maintenance of the local socioeconomic infrastructure and services.

The two types of farms are also complementary in terms of the space that they occupy in the agricultural landscape. Large farms will continue to generate the volume of agricultural produce that fulfills the needs of expanding domestic and export markets. Smaller farms will target niche and local markets while continuing to generate family income through off-farm sources. While large farms will remain highly specialized in their operations, they will integrate numerous subsidiary activities such as transport, handling and processing of farm produce. This has already been anticipated in recent changes to the mandate of Farm Credit Canada which now includes agriculturally-related activities as part of its lending portfolio. Small farms will be more likely to be mixed and engage in pluriactivity operations agri-tourism, etc.

Thus, strategies that focus on the complementary existence of small and large farms would be most beneficial in terms of sustainability, with a respective emphasis on those elements that have the greatest impact on each category.

Characterization of Sustainable Practices Economic

Paying for Sustainability

To be economically viable within the context of

sustainability, Canadian agricultural policy and programs need to shift gears to a third level: the integration of ecological parameters into income support measures. The United States has taken small steps with the conservation measures incorporated into the Farm Bill, and the European Union is taking bigger strides with the integration of environmental measures in the Common Agricultural Policy. Canada is the only industrialized country without a major agricultural conservation program and so it has no choice but to follow.

Farm policy in Canada for the first 100 years was directed at support for the development of food production for an expanding nation. From the free box of seeds and a shovel for every immigrant family willing to take on the task of clearing and cultivating a new farm, through to the crop insurance and farm credit programs, the objective was to make sure that the nation was well fed. The success of these programs, coupled with the advent of the 'green revolution', lead to post-WWII surpluses and the arrival of new orientations geared towards markets - consumers domestically, and for export. Again, from a limited perspective, the marketoriented policies and programs have been a success: Canadian consumers now have access to a much wider range of Canadian-produced foodstuffs, and exports have more than doubled in the last decade.

Success for farmers, especially within the sustainability framework, has been less evident. Despite remarkable achievements in productivity, farm income increases have been modest at best and negative at worst as the 2003 year woefully demonstrated. Even the supply management programs, which have arguably provided dairy and poultry farmers with the most stable and consistent returns in the farming sector, still have not been able to prevent the mass exodus of farmers and provide escape from farm consolidation and production intensification. Every conceivable formulation of income support program has been tried by the federal and provincial governments with little success; even the vaunted income stabilization programs available to Quebec farmers, arguably the best-financed and structured in the country using cost-of-production and return-on-labour formulations, are sometimes assailed as inadequate by the provincial farm organization, the Union des producteurs agricoles.31 The continuing decline in Quebec farm numbers, similar to elsewhere, would support that assertion.

This is not to say that farm income support programs should be abandoned; indeed, given the projected economics of agriculture they will continue to be necessary and, if the principles of sustainable development are adhered to, then there needs to be societal support in order to keep farms economically viable. That being said, however, there is evidently a limit to what governments are prepared to pay, even in disaster situations (BSE-related payments being the latest case in hand), and a lack of political will to maintain subsidies based on production criteria continually and indefinitely.

A new parameter is required, and the integration of environmental factors into the policy and program mix targeting the economic viability of farmers makes more sense:

- There is an emerging and growing recognition that environmental improvements produce a societal benefit for which society should make a contribution towards;
- Environmental payments are de-coupled from production, allowing farmers to produce for the market without distorting influences from income supports;
- Environmental supports are compatible with international trade rules;
- Environmental payments can be made to all types of farms without disadvantage or discrimination, and could be of significant assistance to smaller farms that have lower production volumes;
- Environmental support programs lend themselves well to the emergence and development of 'green' produce

and the opportunity to exploit market opportunities in this regard.

The EU provisions are probably the most comprehensive and far-reaching yet. Although provisions for market and income policy are maintained in the CAP, program payments will only be accessible through cross-compliance measures contained in the section on sustainable development for rural areas . In instances where requirements exceed recognized "good farming practices", additional payments will be made for agri-environmental measures. The program includes specific sub-programs targeted on biodiversity, genetic resources, genetically engineered organisms, climate change (including renewable energy from biomass), soil protection, pesticide use, nitrates, water use and quality, the development of agrienvironmental indicators and forestry.

While similar components of the new CAP approach are present in various Canadian policies and programs, including Agriculture and Agri-Food Canada's Strategy for Sustainable Development, perhaps the biggest challenge to implementing a similar type of program would be federal-provincial jurisdiction. Whereas the EU policy brings individual nations together for a 'common policy', the Canadian system devolves implementation out into 10 provincial jurisdictions, each one with its own set of policies and programs. The decade it has taken to put together a Canadian organic standard stands witness to the monumental task of implementing an effective initiative along the lines of the EU CAP.

This being said, there are a number of opportunities for governments to associate income support with environmental enhancement programs. A coalition of Canadian farm groups has proposed the concept of Alternative Land Use Services, or ALUS.34 This program would provide incentives to agricultural producers to protect wetlands, improve wildlife habitat, conserve riverbank areas and enhance water quality. Another mechanism would be through environmental farm plans which have evolved from a voluntary effort in Ontario supported by the "Green Plan" initiated by the Progressive

Conservative government in the late 1980s, to an integral part of AAFC's Agricultural Policy Framework. EFP allow farmers to develop a comprehensive plan that includes both mandatory reporting requirements (nutrient management plans) and environmental conservation measures. Although the federal government is contributing $48.8 million towards the further uptake of EFPs at the provincial level, these are funds targeted at implementation rather than income support substitution.

Both these programs, and other similar variations, offer the opportunity to support the economic viability of farms while achieving other sustainability goals at the same time. Development of strategies in this regard through AIC would be very timely for Canadian farmers.

Tax on Food

A tax on food is probably a very unpopular proposal with Canadian consumers given that they live in one of the highest taxed nations in the western hemisphere, but they are also the same consumers who enjoy the lowest cost food in the world35 while the people who produce that food are struggling with a substantial drop in income.

Preferably a last resort as a way to raise resources to ensure economic viability for agricultural producers, but a justifiable one none-the-less, such a measure could be implemented as a sales tax on food. Farmers and other social groups fought to exclude food when the GST was enacted in 1991 on the argument that there would be a public backlash and that it was an unjust tax for low-income families given the essential nature of foodstuffs. Sales taxes are now common place, and tax rebate measures have been instituted based on income levels. The 7% GST alone on grocery store sales would generate an estimated $3.3 billion annually, still a considerable sum if only half of it were to be dedicated to supporting economic viability measures for farmers linked to sustainability goals and objectives.

The tax would be efficient to administer given that the

collection system is already in place, and would increase annually along with the rate of inflation and any increase in agri-food imports to ensure an effective and on-going level of support. It would only cost consumers 0.02% of their disposable income which is minimal considering the potential economic and environmental benefits that would accrue.

Biomass for Energy

The promotion of crops for alternate uses (hemp and flax for fiber, corn and grasses for ethanol, and soybeans for biodiesel) has shown potential but has yet to demonstrate returns for farmers. They offer farmers the opportunity to diversify markets and the expectation that shifting commodities over from foodstuffs to energy and fiber will increase demand and therefore prices. They also offer environmental benefits by lowering greenhouse gas emissions and providing farmers with more paying alternatives for crop rotations. Lastly, certain crops, such as switchgrass, are well suited to extensive production on less productive land, thereby increasing revenue from low-output land and keeping it from being intensively cropped.

Safe and Nutritious Food

"One man's meat is another man's poison" is a very apt adage for the current debate around food: is it safe and just how nutritious is it? On the one hand, former federal agriculture minister Lyle Vanclief prefaced the announcement of the discovery of the first case of BSE with the statement that Canada has the safest food system in the world. On the other hand, the Sierra Club of Canada has labeled agriculture as a potential "major threat to the environment" in launching its "Safe Food and Sustainable Agriculture" program.

Food is a complex bundle of personal emotions, family ties, cultural and religious affiliations overlaid by ethical, environmental, political and economic issues. This mix has become volatile as agricultural production, and food processing and distribution, have become more industrialized and ready integrators of new scientific and technological advances. In addition, the consuming public is beginning to suffer from information overload contaminated with the nutrition/diet fad of the week and spiked with propaganda from special interest groups of all stripes.

In a generalized sense, food produced in Canada today is as safe and nutritious as it has ever been, a statement that, no matter how true, becomes meaningless with just one outbreak of salmonella poisoning, one episode of pesticide contamination, or the discovery of just one 'mad cow'. Food safety, as good as it is, lives constantly on the edge, confined by regulation, affected by practice and subject to mishap. The devil is, of course in the details, and although Canada has established a definition of 'safe', the discourse continues at the level of the subsidiary clauses. Safe is defined by the Canadian Food Inspection Agency (CFIA) as a reasonable certainty of no harm while noting that absolute safety cannot be guaranteed and that deliberate study is required to establish whether something is safe in the "broadest sense". The agency also determines that a substance has a history of safe use as a food if it has been an accepted part of the diet for three or more generations in a large, genetically-diverse human population, and used in ways and at levels that are well defined and similar to those expected or intended in the new population. How is it, then, that the relatively new (this generation) introduction of genetically modified corn constitutes a safe product? The current interpretation of 'substantial equivalence' determines that GM corn is the same as conventionallybred corn, and the battle over wording and its interpretation goes from there and has an impact on everything from assessment of novel foods to product labeling.

In this context, this paper cannot delve into, let alone resolve, the many issues revolving around food safety and nutrition; they are far too complex and whole books devoted to the subject have been insufficient to do the same. A more appropriate focus for this paper concerns the issues that can help to resolve some of these debates, those of trust, transparency and understanding. The issue of food safety regulations is covered in a later section on Regulations and Incentives.

Trust

All the declarations of sound science mean little if the public – the mass of individuals who affect policy and regulations through their consumption and voting decisions – do not trust the science. There is little doubt that the public's trust is diminishing with regards to science in general, and there is a loss of confidence in food safety specifically. Even though the human health consequences resulting from the evolution of BSE have, on a relative basis, been uncertain and minimal (not that this in any way diminishes the tragedy of those afflicted by Creutzfeld Jakob Disease), the governmental messages of "It's OK, don't worry" have lacked credibility and undermined the scientific position. This has been further compounded by the dueling debates carried out through the superficial filter of the media ("it's meat… no, it's poison") and the sure and steady transfer of research and development into the commercial arena which, despite its many innovations and achievements, has its own particular biases.

The deterioration of trust regarding the science of food safety has to be reversed and restored to a level that exhibits greater confidence between senders and receivers. This is vital not only on the question of food safety but also for scientific advancement in general – if every new technology gets hooted down simply because there is no trust, society will lose the potential benefits of untold innovations. The case of recombinant Bovine Somatotropin (rBST) in Canada is instructive on this matter: the first applied use of recombinant biotechnology for agricultural production, whatever its merits or misgivings, ended up stalled in Canada due to rampant mistrust throughout the entire approval process. Mistrust of the manufacturer, mistrust of the regulatory process, and mistrust of the science for what has turned out to be a "minor addition to the technology options available to dairy farmers". Some would even argue that, despite the minor overall increase in US milk production resulting from rBST use over the last 11 years, the aggregate effect has been to reduce the number of cows being maintained for production, thus reducing the demand for feed and attendant reductions in the use of water, fuel, and crop inputs. By many standards, such an outcome would be seen as improving the sustainability of agriculture.

There is not one single answer to this question of trust, but evidently it must be tackled through multiple strategies (see following sections on Transparency and Understanding.) One direct approach would be the creation of an independent food authority, perhaps a commissioner's office to provide an arm's length view, and review, of the scientific and regulatory issues related to food safety. This would relieve the Canadian Food Inspection Agency, as it has sometimes been criticized of being both judge and jury when it comes to the approval process for genetically modified crops since it has both a regulatory and promotional role in food safety issues.

Transparency

Many of the issues related to food safety relate to the use of technology – pesticides, antibiotics, biotechnologies – know-how that has been developed, or at least applied, on a commercial basis. Knowledge in these cases has value, and after tens of millions of dollars invested in research, companies are reticent to make that information available to just anyone. This has lead to a situation whereby the approval process is conducted behind closed doors between the applicant and the regulatory authority and, inevitably, that this "lack of transparency in the current approval process leads to an inability to evaluate the scientific rigor of the assessment process, and thus compromises the confidence that society can place in the regulatory framework". See also section "trust" above. Even though this recommendation was made by The Royal Society of Canada Expert Panel on the Future of Food Biotechnology, the suggestion applies equally to all types of technology and processes that have a potential impact on food safety. And rather than being viewed as an additional burden of the regulatory process, it should be regarded as an investment in "sound science" – the peer review and independent verification of research findings that are the foundation principles of the scientific method. The entire debacle concerning transfats could possibly have been avoided if greater scrutiny had been given to addressing the potential for harm that these materials introduced into processed foods. Not only will such an investment result in safe and nutritious food but it will also help greatly to avoid the futile debates that have resulted due to a lack of trust in those who develop and regulate food production and processing technologies. The key question in this regard is what kind of process will accommodate open and rigorous analysis with the need, where appropriate, to maintain proprietary discretion?

Understanding

Questions surrounding food safety and nutrition involve the production, processing and distribution, and consumer components of the agri-food chain. Each is segmented at the regulatory level but the lines blur and the issues meld when viewed as a whole – which is how consumers see the food on their table. This has lead to an unholy mess in terms of how the issues involved in food safety and nutrition are understood, and how that information is acted upon.

A good example is the use of growth hormones in beef production where the popular impression is that feedlot beef are fed buckets-full of the same substances body-builders take to win gold medals – just because they're called steroids. There is little appreciation for the fact that there are many different compositions for hormones and that the amounts present are measured in nanograms (billionths of a gram). One hundred grams of beef coming from a steer treated with a synthetic estrogen-like hormone growth promotant will contain less than 3 nanograms of estrogen; compare that to the 400 nanograms in a serving of peas and the 20,000,000 nanograms present in 100 milliliters of soybean oil and it can be clearly seen that "without such comparative information, consumers are handicapped in choosing the food they eat" (Fairbairn,

1989). The flood of information will only continue to grow as new advances in technology and processing emerge into the agri-food sector, again complicated by the dueling of special interest groups and self-promoters in the mass media. The consequences will not be pretty: as one example, the Atkins Diet, long buried in the backwater obscurity of nutritional fads, rocketed to fame and fortune in 2002 with media-fueled claims of nutritional nirvana for those eating more meat protein over carbohydrates. In August 2005, the company holding the rights to the diet plan declared bankruptcy after suffering a $341 million loss due to slumping demand and competing products. Those who live by the media sword will surely die by the same hand. There are a number of strategies that could be invoked with regard to improving understanding in matters regarding food safety and nutrition, and the AIC, given its mandate and member resources, could be a key player along with other partners.

Agri-food Communications Centre

There is a need for a national centre with a specific focus on communications issues in the agri-food sector. The Food Safety Network46 has been a start as an information resource, as has the SPARK47 program, both located at the University of Guelph. The Farm Credit Corporation has also initiated the "Ag 101 on Highway 1" program for journalism students. While there are web sites and publications that address the importance of food safety and food-borne illness, they are limited and there is a definite lack of data to create an accurate portrait to adequately educate the public about the hazards of unsafe food. Unless an individual is deliberately seeking information concerning food safety, it is unlikely that they will come across the pertinent facts that would be informative about food additives, GMOs, antibiotics or foodborne illnesses. The most common promotion of food safety awareness occurs on fact sheets or FAQ sections within the majority of government and ministry websites and while these are available to the public they are not explicitly evident for educational purposes. It is essential that the consumer have access to accurate, comprehensive and up-to-date information so that they may make educated decisions when purchasing and preparing food.

These types of initiatives need to be built upon and expanded in their range of activities, especially those that include the media and educational programs. Improving access to information is a first step, but this should be followed by training programs for journalists and teachers, as well as support for regional and provincial programs in this regard.

Agri-food in the Classroom

The Agriculture in the Classroom programs are, in principle, a necessary and beneficial activity in promoting understanding about agricultural production. They are, however, limited by a crowded academic agenda and minimal access for the overwhelmingly urban clientele to farms and agri-food facilities. These programs need to be supported beyond their current ad hoc and under-resourced status, but they also need to be expanded to include what used to be called home economics. Re-introducing cooking into the school curriculum would not only provide important life skills beyond the capacity to microwave a frozen dinner, it would also present the opportunity to broaden the knowledge and understanding of students and teachers about food – and what makes it safe and nutritious. This could certainly be included within the mandate of the Agricultural Communications Centre as well.

There are also a number of *PATs* (pay attention to's) that require some consideration within the context of sustainability and food safetynutrition.

Traceability

The capacity to track any morsel of food back to its point of origin has become, to some extent, the holy grail of food safety policies and programs. While this capability is recognized by all, including farmers, as an essential component in safeguarding the modern agri-food system, it also risks undermining one of the important tenats of sustainability –

small farms – which are beginning to drown in paperwork that literally requires filing forms when moving livestock from one pasture to another. As with all government programs, farmers need some elements of practicality in their implementation which will require differentiation related to farm size, even separate systems adapted to local markets.49

Nutrition

On any given produce container found on today's supermarket shelves, consumers can find more information about the contents than they care to digest. Information, however, does not equate with understanding, and it is a question worth posing just how much understanding is fostered through the placement of truncated values in miniscule font on the back of soup cans. The utilization of modern information technology seems to be an appropriate solution in that very detailed information regarding the general elements of nutrition and the specific attributes of a given item could be key coded into a database and made available from a terminal at the point of purchase (scan the bar code and up comes that product's information), and also on the Internet. Such a mechanism would also help promote understanding about fresh fruits and vegetables. A common claim is that organic tomatoes taste better than conventionally-produced ones; it isn't because the tomatoes are organic, it's because the conventional tomatoes are picked green before they ripen to prevent damage during transportation and therefore have less sugar in the fruit when finally stimulated to turn red through ethylene gasification.

MPI

The crop sector has developed IPM, or integrated pest management, as a strategy to minimize the use of synthetic inputs in the production of a particular commodity. With regard to food safety and nutrition, this acronym needs to be flipped with the developed of strategies for MPI – minimal process interference. MPI could become an indicator of sustainability by showing just how far evolved a particular food product is from its natural state, including the use of crop protection materials, processing changes and additions, and packaging and distribution. An untreated apple plucked from a tree scores a 10, baked goods made with transfats ends up way down the list. A tricky process to develop such an indicator, but no doubt a stimulus to move towards more sustainable production practices.

Star Trek Menu

Despite rapid advances in food technology, we are still a long way off from the type of computerized 'food' generators popularized in the Star Trek television series. But the 'disassembly' of whole foods into constituent parts has been underway for sometime, and is now beginning to move forward into the molecular realm. Corn is no longer grown just for the kernel but for the starches and oils – both indigenous and modified – that are segregated and reassembled as something else, and nanoscience will take this even further with the ability to synthesize proteins and other molecular substances; this will have significant bearing on the application of definitions such as substantial equivalence and novel foods.50 Such capacity has huge implications for questions of sustainability, and although there are no ready answers now, leaving the debate until after these products hit the supermarket shelves will be an abdication of the scientific discourse.

Vibrant Rural Communities

Worldwide, there is at least one consistent pattern amongst human societies: the movement of populations from the countryside to the cities. Whether it is Mexico, India or South Africa, populations are heading toward the urban centers, driven by socio-political pressures and in search of a perceived better life. The further the rural region is away from a predominant urban concentration, the more this appears to be the case. In Canada, rural residents are abandoning the farthest points of rural regions to add to the immigrantfueled expansion of major cities and adjacent corridors: Quebec City-

Windsor, Calgary-Edmonton, and Vancouver-Fraser Valley.

The history of much of rural Canada since settlement by European immigrants is synonymous with farming, and farmers made up us much as 31.7% of the Canadian population in 193151, and a much greater proportion of the rural population as well. Today, the farm population numbers sit at less than 2.4% of total population (2001 census), and an average of only 11.5% of the rural population, which itself is declining as a percentage of total population.52 In this context, many rural communities once made 'vibrant' by their farm population are struggling with fewer employment opportunities, school and hospital closings and an aging population. Within the parameters of sustainable agriculture, the literature repeatedly lays the blame for this situation on some combination of large corporate industrialized farms, along with an attendant claim that going back to having more small farms will resolve the situation for rural communities. While it is true that large corporate industrialized farms have come to dominate the farming landscape, is it true that they are the cause or really just the outcome? The single largest decline in farm numbers occurred in the decade up to 1961, the same period when most farms became electrified and tractors, along with useful adjuncts such as hydraulics, replaced horses as the main source of agri-production power.53 Another example of this parameter are the supply managed farms which, despite being afforded the most border protection of all Canadian commodities from the negative affects of freer trade, have not been able to escape from a similar decline in farm numbers.

Numerous studies have demonstrated that more small farms can make an overall greater contribution to rural community vitality than fewer large farms; this only stands to reason given that there would be more people present in the particular location. But without massive state intervention the resurrection of many more small farms is unlikely to happen given that small farms are (in a general sense and in the current context) not economically viable, spending as much as $1.68

in operating expenses in order to take in one dollar of receipts.55 Rather than looking at strategies to specifically increase the number of small farms, the approach should be to look at ways in which agriculture can make a contribution to the vibrancy of rural communities, big farm or small.

Owner/operator

One of the most frequent references to the detrimental affects of large farms to the life of rural communities is the use of the term "corporate". Certainly rural communities, and agriculture itself, have lots to fear from non-farming corporations owning and operating agricultural production capacity in order to ensure supply and quality parameters for the processing and distribution ends of the agri-food chain, especially when this is carried out at a loss in order to make larger profits further downstream. As a reminder of where this can lead, in the United States, 110 farms representing 0.18% of the total number of hog farms, holds 54% of livestock inventory in this sector.

If current trends continue, more and more farms will become incorporated as they grow in size, which will simply reflect appropriate management strategies rather than any conspiracy of corporate concentration. The key element for sustainability will be to develop a framework whereby policies and programs favour the operation of the farm by the owner(s), a term that would, by necessity, include local farm operators with land ownership and or long-term leasing arrangements. Operation by local ownership, regardless of farm structure, would ensure greater socio-economic commitment to the local community by larger farms (based on the same assumptions for small farms that local presence brings benefit), as well as more extensive engagement in environmental conservation.

No doubt such a strategy will entail considerable debate in order to define practical application, but it will be much more useful than to continue using such terms as "large" or "corporate". It may be difficult to mandate an 'owner/ operator' status by regulation, but would certainly be achievable through policy and program approaches encouraging such a status, for example by restricting access to income supports.

Value Added

It's become a bit of a cliché to say that "adding value" beyond the farm gate will act as a panacea for all that ails the economics of agriculture. There is no doubt, however, that the presence of a local post-production processing and/or distribution facility creates employment and economic development opportunities. Even though farm employment has declined, employment in the agri-food sector past the farm gate has grown faster than the overall economy , an indicator that there is value to be had for rural communities when agricultural production is combined with locally situated processing and distribution activities.

Strategic Alliances

Strategic alliances may be just another cliché, but nonetheless the concept is appropriate in this context. The predominant macro-trend in the agri-food sector is concentration - fewer and bigger farms, processors and retailers - and little in the way of policies or programs seems to be making a difference in this regard. Farmers have tended to stay as individuals (even as members of collective structures such as co-operatives, or in direct contractual relationships such as integration) and therefore remain less capable of resisting the 'get big or get out' syndrome.

The notion of exchange and/or co-operation between farmers in order to provide greater critical mass in terms of production and processing capacity i.e. custom combining, livestock transport has been part of farm operations and management for the longest time. There appear to be benefits that can accrue by expanding the range of these types of working relationships between farmers on a strategic basis in order to maintain farm numbers while providing benefits from economies of scale. Luc Robitaille, of Mont-St-Gregoire,

Quebec, was one of the farmers interviewed for this paper. He owns a typical Quebec hog farm with 1,500 acres of crop land providing feed for 5,000 feeder hogs and 1200 sows.

He is, however, the pivot man for 57 other farms connected through strategic alliances that includes a further 10,000 acres of crops, a feed mill processing 180,000 tonnes of grain a year and an abattoir that slaughters 4,000 hogs a week, in addition to the sharing of a multitude of technical and professional resources. Some of the participating farms have shares in the various operations, some just purchase services, and others have contracts – each unto their own.

Farm Succession

A typical policy recommendation from farm groups is that farm succession, or intergenerational transfers, must be facilitated if there is going to be a next generation of farmers in Canada.58 An aging farm population and an exit rate, if left unchanged, will reduce the number of Canadian farmers to less than 150,000 farms by 2021, which means that encouraging and facilitating farm transfers will be a critical aspect of sustaining agriculture. It is a daunting task given that in Quebec, even though a young farmer has support from a stabilized or supply managed income based on cost-of-production formulas, access to subsidized farm credit and a start-up grant as much as $40,000 depending on the level of post-secondary education, farm numbers are declining on par with other provinces.

The easy answer is to make farming more economically attractive, but in the meantime there are a number of strategies that might be pursued:

Fiscal

Both federal and provincial governments have, over the last two decades or so, progressively removed many of the fiscal incentives that made the 'cash poor, paper rich' nature of farming viable. The zeal of tax departments to ensure that absolutely no city doctor or lawyer receives any tax advantage from operating their country estate as a farm has left bona fide young farmers bereft of most of the former fiscal enticements their parents enjoyed being able to deduct house taxes and electricity consumption against income tax were not huge amounts but were sufficient to assist in farm start-ups and low income years. Rejuvenated fiscal strategies would be welcome support for encouraging young farmers.

Non-farming Farmers

The success rate of converting non-farmers to the farming way of life has been mixed, and it is to be expected that engaging in full ownership of a farm with little experience and or training is not a recipe for high rates of achievement. However, if there is to be an infusion of new blood in the agriculture sector, then many of those prospective participants will have to come from non-farming backgrounds. Throwing them cold turkey into farming situations is no more likely to result in success than before; establishing training and employment opportunities targeted at skilled agricultural workers will allow new job participants to acquire experience in the sector while assisting larger farms through the provision of an improved labour pool. New programs to facilitate partial farm ownership or share cropping, such as is commonly done with dairy herd milkers in New Zealand, would be a further incentive for re-engagement in agriculture and, therefore, rural communities.

Immigration

Canada is a country that was founded on immigration and continues to grow through an influx of new arrivals in the 21st Century few of whom choose to settle in rural communities. There are many possibilities to encourage immigration into rural communities, but they all require some change in government policies and programs to come about; some suggestions are:

- More flexible provisions for professionals (doctors, teachers, etc.) to be able to work much sooner after arrival on condition they take up placement in rural locations for a designated period; this would also improve the social infrastructure for rural communities, which is also a contributing factor to exodus.

Allowance for seasonal workers brought in from other countries to become landed immigrants after several years of engagement on that basis;

Development of social structures to assist new arrivals, such as community-owned or cooperative housing, that provides them with some stability for their new family life.

Conservation of Resources and Environment

Agriculture is one of the biggest users of 'space' amongst the different economic sectors in Canada, occupying some 68 million hectares of land mass across the country, 61% of which is cultivated.60 Add in to that expanse the increasingly intensive production methods of the last 50 years and the fact that large segments of agricultural land is located near urban populations, and agriculture has resulted in some negative impacts on the environment as well as being a major consumer of off-farm resources. Much attention has been paid to the environmental impact of agriculture in the last 20 years, and, as a consequence, a variety of policies, programs, and regulations have been developed and put into place - such as water protection policies, environmental farm plans and nutrient management plans. Some have targeted containment (strategies to reduce pollution), others have focused on management practices, and yet others have highlighted the need to raise awareness levels. The two main criteria used to judge the environmental sustainability for agriculture are how well the natural resources that support agricultural production are managed and conserved, and how compatible agricultural systems are with natural systems and processes.

This can be done, and in so doing helping to minimize negative environmental impacts, by assessing agricultural operations in terms of their environmental risk and then managing and developing them to minimize that risk.62 This strategy implies three assumptions:

- that the correct aspects of the farm are being assessed;
- that the assessment is as accurate as possible; and
- that the farmer is able to implement the necessary changes (as well as maintain current practices where no changes are required.)

The five major aspects of the farm which should be evaluated, acted upon and monitored are

- livestock facilities and infrastructure
- land nutrient management (including manure, fertilizer and other soil amendments)
- soil erosion
- energy efficiency
- biodiversity

The anticipated results that should be obtained once any necessary changes have been implemented, and the practices that are most likely to achieve them, are shown in the following table.

Expected results once practices or changes implemented

- All facilities should be leakage free
- Tolerable but minimal odour and dust
- Application of nutrients from manure and other sources to meet crop needs while maintaining optimal crop yields and soil fertility
- Method and timing of application and speed of incorporation to minimize the risk of nutrient run-off and leaching.

- Soil erosion is reduced to a level where soil productivity can be maintained for the foreseeable future
- Soil erosion is reduced to a level where its impact on water quality in permanent watercourses does not prevent the water from meeting current standards for maximal usage
- The farm generates true carbon credits
- The energy efficiencies achieved are at least such that if the harvested biomass from a farm was to be converted into ethanol, the amount of energy in the ethanol would exceed the energy expenditure used for the production, transport and treatment of the raw biomass.
- Wetlands, highly sensitive lands, forested lands that are inadequate for agriculture are protected
- Watercourses used as a corridor for both wildlife shelter and restored as routes for animal migration

Best practices to achieve results

- Water tight and certified manure storage
- Filter strips fields around potential sources of contaminated water such as leachates from bunker silos and run-off from outside yards
- Windbreaks around facilities, placed on the side of the dominant wind.
- Application and incorporation of nutrients should be such that:
- the mineralization of nutrients and crop uptake are synchronized and therefore both the inorganic content of the material and the C/N ratio should be taken into account when deciding timing for application and incorporation

- the application of nutrients should not compromise the physical health of the soil and therefore soil moisture content should be taken into account when deciding timing for application.

Watershed Management

Watercourses are a neutral and common space shared between agriculture and other segments of society. The watercourses are not developed or used in the same sense as land, yet they are important to all who occupy their borders. They have also become a flashpoint for environmental conflicts between farmers and surrounding rural residents as well as downstream urban populations. Much of this revolves around who is responsible for what portion of environmental damage when there is non-point source pollution from agriculture as well as point source pollution from industry, municipal sewage and residential septic systems. Management by watershed objectives enables the participation of all interested stakeholders, the establishment of benchmarks and the measurement of site-specific improvements.

Windbreaks

Although manure receives most of the bad rap for non-point source pollution, soil erosion is much more of a culprit given that the movement of soil particles from the fields carries potential pollutants along with them.66 Soil erosion is a major pathway by which nutrients and other pollutants reach watercourses. A lot of progress has been made in this regard through best management practices that prevent excessive water run-off and leaching, as well as the reduction in airborne erosion through minimum tillage practices. Further improvement can be achieved through the establishment of windbreaks which have the added benefit of diversifying habitat. While windbreaks are often in conflict with the size of modern machinery, programs to target the most sensitive areas would contribute significantly to soil erosion reduction and riverbank stabilization.

Energy

It will probably be the most unpopular statement in this paper, but the higher the cost of fossil fuel energy goes, the better it will be for the sustainability of agriculture. The era where the demand for energy is exceeding conventional supplies is upon us and all sectors of society will be forced to reconsider their energy sources and the way it is consumed.

A great deal of work has already begun on the role of agriculture in contributing to the reduction of global warming by reducing the production of greenhouse gasses, and increasing the sequestration of carbon in the soil. These are potential sources of revenue or tax credits, but will require further assessment of current levels of energy efficiency and the implementation of energy efficient farming practices.

Roles and Potential Impacts Research and Extension

One of the fundamental pillars of agricultural development in North America has been the research and extension network, particularly in the United States where a series of federal laws enacted starting in 1862 lead to the creation of the land grant university system that joined with state-run cooperative extension networks to serve the farm and rural populations. The applied research results taught to university students and transferred to the agricultural sector through outreach programs can arguably be cited as one of the most important investments in the development of the world's most productive agricultural nation. Canada has instituted some variations to the land grant/cooperative extension model, institutions and services that have been developed on a less consistent and pervasive basis than in the US, and one that has now "decreased significantly due to declining resources". Typical of the situation is specialization of research facilities, with research itself becoming more market driven and intellectual property and patenting issues restricting the dissemination of research. This is of particular concern to the progression of sustainability in agriculture because there is a need for systems information - knowledge - rather than just new applied technologies, and those applied technologies required within the context of sustainability seem to have less commercial appeal for the current system of development. Where are the drought resistant or less fertilizer dependent crop varieties that have been part of the promise of biotechnology for some years?

There are numerous studies and reports in recent years that provide many good suggestions on actions to be taken with regard to agricultural research and extension which includes the notion of technology transfer. Unfortunately, many of these suggestions include the phrase "the government should" which, given the retreat by both federal and provincial governments from fully-funded programs in these areas over the last two decades, is not going to move the agricultural sustainability agenda very fast. Following are some suggestions to get things moving a little faster.

Research Levy

A levy on commodities is one way to inject sufficient funds to expand in the short-term research and extension efforts on sustainable agricultural practices. This will obviously not be popular with farmers given that research and extension services have largely been provided at little cost to farmers to date, but it should be viewed as an investment that will return dividends through improved margins. A commodity levy will have the benefit of allowing farmers to direct research according to their needs, especially for on-farm research, and allow them to access existing government programs which are mostly allocated on a matching fund basis. The government can make a contribution to the research/extension agenda through the provision of fiscal incentives to ensure that there is longer term stability in the network.

Producer-operated Extension Structures

The general demise of a uniform (at least at the provincial level) and state-run extension network has left in its place an ad hoc network of programs, services, organizations and institutions providing information and services to farmers. This means that some farmers, particularly the furthest away, lack service, and that some services are more targeted towards, and accessible by, larger farms. In addition, an increasing amount of information and service provided to farmers is through farm suppliers even though it is not necessarily the preferred source.

As with research, it is unlikely that the existing extension services will be resurrected to their former state, or expanded beyond where they currently exist. As much as extension-type information was important in the past, it will be equally important in the future as the pace of scientific knowledge and technological innovation continues unabated. There is, in this context, the need for new structures to ensure that extension services are available to all farmers on an unconditional basis. Already some interesting models have emerged, from soil and crop associations in some provinces, to the producer clubs and centers of expertise in Quebec. The role and place of these structures needs to be refined and expanded given that they are a particularly important mechanism for supporting and serving smaller-sized farms.

Information Technologies

Agriculture benefited enormously from the introduction of electricity which was accomplished in a relatively rapid time span through public policy initiatives that aimed to provide all Canadians with access to service on an equitable basis. The same can be said about early telecommunications in rural areas, such as radio and telephone. Not so in the modern information era: there are still some rural residents, farmers amongst them, who cannot operate a fax machine because they are still on a party line. The knowledge economy is far removed from many of these communities because the upgrade in infrastructure required for the provision of hi-speed Internet and the like will occur sometime. The deregulation of the telecommunications sector, from a rural perspective, has been a tremendous disservice and a failure of public policy to support the development of non-urban areas at a time when the relative benefit of new technologies could have much more impact given the greater distances and dispersed locations that are characteristic of service provision in the regions. There needs to be the creation of programs and provisions that allow the comprehensive uptake of advances in information technologies in rural areas within much shorter time frames after their introduction in urban markets. This will either require compensatory resources from public funds, or provisions that facilitate and support local telecommunications initiatives over the longer term.

Incentives, Regulations and Indicators

Environment

In the past few years the implementation of environmentally friendly farming models and practices have been driven by a mixture of regulations, incentives, education, and personal values. It is clear however that regulations and incentives are the most effective way to achieve rapid change on a large scale. In North America, a number of regional governments have adopted a mixture of regulations and incentives to compel farmers into changing their practices in order to minimize the environmental impact. These packages come in various combinations, which impose constraints on farming practices, and sometimes the regulations must be met in order to have access to government programs – this is often referred to as "eco-compliance", or "éco-conditionnalité" in Quebec. Other programs offer payments for setting aside farm land in order to protect marginal types of land or create buffer zones next to fragile bordering areas. On occasion, programs have made payments for the adoption of specific cultural practices such as planting cover crops for winter periods.

This brings about two consequences for farmers. The first is that they must adopt environmentally friendly farming practices that are defined by the regulations. Because the farm is a system, changes to one aspect of the farm's management will affect other aspects of the farm. For example, it might be necessary to apply liquid hog manure in the spring to avoid late fall application which has become restricted by regulation in some areas. This requires better spreading equipment to avoid soil compaction and the addition of increased storage capacity for the manure. It also impacts on the time available for planting, and the choice of crops. The second consequence is that the farmer must be able to monitor what is being done, and to complete the paper work in order to be able to produce a trail for auditing and monitoring. Even though much of the paper work is handled by professional agronomists and technicians, the farm manager must still be aware of the implications in order to be able to make effective management decisions. In this regard, the farm manager must have the ability to control the bureaucratic aspects of the regulations as they apply to the farm.

Both these effects put pressure on individual farm systems, and on the farming community as a whole. It also tends to wean out of agriculture the farms that are not able to meet the regulatory constraints (assuming that they are environmentally 'unfriendly'), but also the farms which are unable to adapt to the imposition of the regulations and the bureaucratic burden that comes with them. This has raised a major issue with farmers in that measures to make farms more environmentally sustainable are, at the same time, stimulating some farmers to exit the sector.

The farms that are most likely to be able to meet the regulatory constraints and survive the paper work requirements are likely to be those with more resources at their disposal (often larger farms) and higher levels of management skills. These farms have more capacity and depth to handle the increasing demands with regard to agri-environmental management. Consequently, the imposition of a regulatory framework regarding sustainable agriculture is likely to further accelerate the trend towards bigger farms.

Variable Regulations

In one respect, this is the direction that has already been taken by most regional governments. The regulations tend to leave out the very small farms and phase in farms over time according to their size, the bigger and newer farm operations being targeted first. This gives more time for smaller farms to comply with environmental constraints.

However, the regulations are not modulated according to the size of the farm, that is to say that every farm that has to comply, has to comply with the same regulations. An extensive cow-calf operation with 50 animal units located away from any permanent watercourse with an effective land use to animal unit ratio of more than 2:1 has to face the same regulatory burden as an intensive hog or poultry farm in an opposite situation. This 'one size fits all' characteristic appears to have more to do with matching regulations to available government monitoring resources than with the effective agri-environmental management of the particular farming operation.

More Management

So far, efforts by governments in terms of monitoring, and by farmers in terms of adopting new practices, have been implemented using a variety of models and with different levels of emphasis. It is still unclear, however, whether these efforts have resulted in the expected outcomes as far as environmental quality is concerned. One of the weaknesses of the current approach is that the monitoring of change implementation, and the consequent effects, lags behind the assessment and recommendation stages. In other words, when a farmer makes a plan and complies with government standards, the follow-up on the implementation of the changes included in the plan and their impact on the environment is inadequate or missing entirely. In effect, there is a significant amount of resource being dedicated to regulatory compliance with less focus on the monitoring of the impact or outcome, and with little purposeful integration of the regulatory measures within the management regime of the farm. The 'Bilan phosphore' (soil phosphorus level report) in Quebec, and similar mechanisms in some other provinces, is a regulatory requirement linked to eco-compliance beyond which there is no environmental management component – as long as farmers file the report to demonstrate that their land does not exceed threshold levels, they are deemed to be in compliance. Sustainable agricultural practices within the regulatory context could be advanced through the development of strategies that support variable applicability (on a farm-by-farm basis) and integration of environmental management aspects in conjunction with the regulatory framework. The movement toward individual environmental farm plans is an example of one such strategy.

Incentives

While regulations set the framework, incentives are the positive reinforcement that gets things moving. The case of the Watershed Agricultural Council in New York state is a prime example. The organization has negotiated a 'fee-for-service' arrangement with New York City for providing clean water in the Hudson River watershed which provides the city with its drinking water. The funds permit the Council to pay farmers and foresters to implement practices that ensure clean upstream water, such as set asides and buffer zones along feeder tributaries. The city pays for these services as a preventative measure that reduces their costs for water treatment. Farmers have been advocating for support for the multifunctional nature of agriculture, and the identification of opportunities whereby farmers can be compensated for providing a service would greatly assist in the incorporation of sustainable practices within farming operations.

Safe and Nutritious Food

A very sophisticated and comprehensive set of auditing, monitoring and certification systems are being put in place through the agri-food chain to meet the growing demands to ensure that food is safe and nutritious. The Hazard Analysis Critical Control Point Safety Enhancement Program Canadian On-Farm Food Safety Program as well as organic certification, regional product identification etc. are all examples of this activity at different levels. The concern with systems such as these is not that they will not ensure food safety and nutrition, but that they could lead to complacency that additional monitoring methods can be developed *ad infinitum* to cover new forms of food production or processing. Is there any limit to the number of critical control points within the concept of sustainability? Considerable reflection must be given to just how much monitoring systems can do in terms of producing safe food in a sustainable manner. Part of this comes back to the notion of minimal process intervention, and part of it comes back to the burden that small farms and small agri-food enterprises face in complying to yet another set of standards. There is no end to the list of items that may be considered in terms of strategies to advance the sustainability of Canadian agriculture. Some fit in with common categories, such as with the approaches to environmental conservation already mentioned in this paper. There are others, however, that are less suited to categorization but still worth giving some thought to.

Bibliography

Anderson, A.J., 'The Role of Molybdenum in Plant Nutrition', *Inorganic Nitrogen Metabolism*, Ed., Mick Elroy, W.D., and Glass, B. (The Johns Hopkins Press, Baltimore, 1956).

Bergel, F., *Chemistry of Enzymes in Cancer* (Charles C. Thomas, Springfield, Ill. U.S.A., 1961).

Beyers, E., 'Treatment of Mineral Deficiencies', *The Deciduous Fruit Grower* (June 1954).

Brown, J.C. and Tiffin, L.O., 'Properties of Chelates and Their Use In Crop Production', *Agri. Food Chem.*, **10**, 192-195 (1962).

Caskey, C.D. and Norris, L.C., 'Further Studies on the Roles on Manganese in Poultry Nutrition', *Poult. Sci.*, **17**, 433 (1938).

Chenoweth, M.B., "Chelation as a Mechanism of Pharmaçological Action", *Pharmacol Reb.*, **8**, 57-87 (1956).

Davis, G.K., 'Metabolic Function and Practical Use of Cobalt in Nutrition', *Trace Elements*, ed. LAMB, C.A., and Beattie, J.M. (Academic Press, New York and London, 1958).

Hewitt, E. J. and McCready, C.C., 'Relation of Nitrogen Supply to the Molybdenum Requirement of Tomato Plants Grown in Sand Culture', Nature, 174, 186-7 (1954).

Koehler, F. E., and Albrecht, W.A., 'Biosynthesis of Amino Acids According to Soil Fertility, III, Bioassays of Forage and Grain Fertilized with Trace Elements', *Plant & Soil*, **4**, 336-44 (1953).

Lee, H. J., 'The Toxicity of *Phalaris tuberosa* to Sheep and Cattle, and the Preventive Role of Cobalt', *Proc. VII. Int Grassld. Congr., Wellington, N.Z.*, 387-96 (1956).

Mulder, E. G., 'The Essentiality of Trace Elements for Microorganisms and the Microbiological Determination of these Elements', *Atti del VI Congresso Internat. Di Microbiologia, Roma,* **6** (No. 18), 293-313 (1953).

Mulder, E. G., 'Trace Element Conditions in Relation to Soil Conditions', *Pontif. Acad. Sci. Scripta Varia,* **14,** 215-232 (1954).

Plumlee, M. P., Thrasher, D. M., Beeson, W. M., Andrews, F. N., and Parker, H.e., 'The Effects of Manganese Deficiency upon the Growth, Development and Reproduction of Swine', *J. Animal Sci.,* **15,** 352-367 (1956).

Polukhina, I. N., and Masljanaja, H.K., ' Influence of Nitrogen and Copper on the Anatomical Structure of Oat Stems in Relation to the Resistance of Oats on Peat Soils' (English translation), *Izv. Timit. Sol. Shokh Akad.,* No. 1, 205-208 (1961).

SchÜtte, K. H., and Schendel, H. E., 'Effect of Trace Elements on Plant Protein Composition', *Proc. Nutr. Soc. S. A.,* 2, 47-50 (1961).

STOCKS, P., and DAVIS, R. I., 'Epidemiological Evidence from Cemical and Spectographic Analysis that the Soil is Concerned in the Causation of Cancer', *Brit J. Cancer',* 14, 8-23 (1960).

Stookey, G. K. Crane, D. B. and Muhler, J. C. 'Effect of Molybdenum on Fluoride Absorption', *Proc. Soc. exp Biol. Med,* 109, 580-583 (1962).

Timberlake, C. F., 'Complex Formation between Copper and Some Organic Acids, Phenols and Phenolic Acids Occurring in Fruit', J. Chem. Soc., 2795-2798 (1959).

Zimmerman, P. W., and Hitchcock, A.E., 'Susceptibility of Plants to Hydrofluoric Acid and Sulphur Dioxide Gases', *Contrib. from Boyce Thompson Instit.,* 18, 263-279 (1955).

Index